From CP to CPA:

One Man's Triumph over the Disability of Cerebral Pasly

How one man "shook" down the barriers along life's pathways and overcame a crippling disability to achieve his personal dreams-and how you can too.

Robin Pritts

From CP to CPA:

One Man's Triumph over the Disability of Cerebral Palsy

ISBN: 0-9722719-3-7

Copyright © 2002 Robin Pritts

All rights reserved. No part of this publication may be reproduced, stored in a retrieval system, or transmitted in any form or any other means electronic, mechanical, photocopying, recording or otherwise, without the prior written permission of the publisher.

Author photo courtesy of Cherie Wayne (www.cheriewayne.com)
Cover and interior design: Weyant Press Design
Cover design elements: royalty-free clipart

Published in the United States by

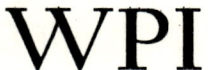

Weyant Press, Inc.
Success Series Division

27765 McKee Road
Toney, Alabama 35773
www.weyantpress.com

In Praise of

FROM CP TO CPA:
One Man's Triumph over the Disability of Cerebral Palsy

"What a precious gift Robin has given us in sharing the often heartrending lessons he's learned in his short life! Not only is he an extraordinary man with extraordinary courage, but he also helps us realize that we, too, can be extraordinary, no matter what our disability may be. Robin gave me a wake-up call--to stop whining about the things going wrong in my life and instead, to focus on all the blessings I've received. Thank you, Robin, for sharing your heart in such an open and honest way. We will all be better people for having read your book."
-**Barbara Glanz, CSP**, Author of *CARE Packages for the Home* and *CARE Packages for the Workplace*

"Robins book, From CP to CPA is not only empowering for physically challenged people but for all ! I am totally blessed that I can wake up each day and know that I have shared a brief moment in history with a man named Robin Pritts."
-**Philippe Matthews**, Author *How To Make Millions When Thousands Have Been Laid Off*

"Mr. Pritts . . . draws upon his sum of experiences to motivate, challenge, and inform his audience."
-**Dr. Matthew Wanzenberg**, *Aurora University Instructor*

"Listening to Rob is always a uniquely rewarding experience."
-**Steve Schroeder**, *Director of Forensics, College of DuPage*

DEDICATION:

I want to dedicate this book to "My Loving Families." (I have had three or four special groups, besides my real family, who have made a difference in my life; I think you know who you are.) I would also like to dedicate it to my friends. Without the help of these dear people, friends and families alike, I would never have made it this far.

Thank you, each and every one, for your unconditional love, support, and inspiration . . .

TABLE OF CONTENTS:

FOREWORD: *Transforming Barriers into Opportunities by Maureen N. Dunne*

INTRODUCTION: WE ARE ALL DISABLED	1
SECTION ONE: BARRIERS IN YOUR PATH	3
BARRIERS PLACED THERE BY OTHERS	9
ENVISION THE POSSIBILITIES	11
WORKING WITH THE SYSTEM	17
PICKING YOUR BATTLES	23
AVOIDING PITY PARTIES	29
BARRIERS PLACED THERE BY YOURSELF	33
QUITTING IS NOT AN OPTION!	35
YOUR DISABILITY IS NOT AN EXCUSE	41
(NOT) MAKING THE GRADE	47
YOUR ATTITUDE DETERMINES YOUR ALTITUDE	51
MAKE PLANS, NOT WISHES	59
SECTION TWO: UNDERSTANDING THE PATH	63
UNDERSTANDING OTHERS	67
ACCENTUATE THE POSITIVE	69
ADAPTING BEFORE IT WAS MANDATED	73
DEALING WITH MISUNDERSTANDING	77
FIGHTING STEREOTYPES	81
DON'T EXPECT RESPECT-UNTIL YOU EARN IT!	85
UNDERSTANDING YOURSELF	89
BE CAREFUL WHAT YOU WISH FOR . . .	91
DON'T BLAME YOUR DISABILITY	95
DON'T CONFUSE A CHANCE WITH A RISK	99
GIVING TO RECEIVE	103
PUTTING YOUR DISABILITY INTO PERSPECTIVE	107

SECTION THREE: QUAKE THE BARRIERS — 111

WITH THE HELP OF OTHERS — 115
    SEEKING INSPIRATION FROM INSPIRING TEACHERS — 117
    VALUING FRIENDSHIP — 121
    NEVER LOSE FAITH IN YOUR FELLOW MAN — 125
    LEARN TO EXCEL WHERE YOU FEEL MOST COMFORTABLE — 131

BY YOURSELF — 129
    NEVER GIVE UP HOPE — 137
    BE A FRIEND TO YOURSELF FIRST — 141
    PUT YOURSELF IN THE PATH OF LIFE'S LITTLE SURPRISES — 145
    MOST LIKELY TO SUCCEED — 149
    ALWAYS WANT MORE — 153
    PUTTING YOUR TRUST IN PROFESSIONALS — 157

CONCLUSION: *HONING YOUR SKILLS (FOR LIFE)!* — 161

AFTERWORD: *What's Next?* — 167

FOREWORD:

Transforming Barriers Into Opportunities
by Maureen N. Dunne

From CP to CPA: One Man's Triumph Over the Disability of Cerebral Palsy is an inspiring book that illuminates a central theme: However difficult the circumstances, one can successfully navigate through barriers to achieve his or her personal and professional goals. As a child, the author, Robin Pritts, was diagnosed with Cerebral Palsy. Cerebral Palsy, a condition that affects control of the muscles, however, has not prevented Rob from excelling at the University of Illinois, becoming a certified public accountant, nor succeeding as an inspiring motivational speaker.

Drawing upon three decades of wisdom and experience, Rob shares some of his most challenging moments, and perhaps more importantly, how he managed them. In doing so, he transforms disability into difference and barriers into opportunities. Rather than focus on his own disability, Rob challenges others to conceptualize the world as "disabled" and offers many fresh insights. As a way of bridging the gap between the disabled and non-disabled worlds, Rob reminds us that "whether it is shaking or being too short to reach the top shelf in the kitchen, we are all saddled with disabilities that we need to overcome," (p. 4).

Moreover, by illustrating how he has succeeded personally and professionally despite disability, Rob advises others to continue along their path even when faced with difficulties and adversity. Further, according to Rob, it is only by acknowledging the ineffectiveness of an "us" versus "them" attitude and building upon the strengths of all individuals, whether labeled disabled or non-disabled, that progress can be achieved.

By sharing his journey, Rob invites the reader to rethink assumptions about persons with disabilities and provides sound advice to get through life's challenges. In Rob's own words, "It's how we react to those disabilities, it's how we break down the barriers they present, or work our way around them, over them, or through them, that determines how big or little those disabilities are," (p. 4).

Persons with disabilities, as well as parents, family, and friends, will likely find Rob's story both inspiring and helpful as they are learning to navigate through their own personal barriers. Educators will also find this book invaluable as it provides an insider view of a former special education student whom successfully navigated the system to achieve his high academic and personal goals. From CP to CPA not only contains encouraging advice for the general population, but additionally furthers the aims of the disability movement.

-Maureen N. Dunne, Rhodes Scholar, Division on Medical Sciences, Oxford University, England

INTRODUCTION:

We are All Disabled

The worlds of the disabled and the "normal" often cross paths-and not always pleasantly. But just think how much better we'd get along if we ALL thought of ourselves as disabled . . .

Like the rest of the world, I have to deal with my strengths and weaknesses in my own unique manner. Many people look at the accomplishments I have managed to achieve in my short life and are amazed that someone who is disabled could have done so much.

Yet I am constantly thinking of how much more there is to do! And if I sat around and spent all of my precious time labeling myself with words like "disabled" and "handicapped," I'd be too busy to ever do anything productive. That is why I say that, in a way, we are ALL disabled. But how?

Don't we all have some area in which we need help? What about the computer illiterate, who panics every time his laptop makes a noise, opens an extra window, sends him an "error" message, crashes, or freezes up? In today's technological age, this is definitely a disability that is likely to affect his job performance, his level of proficiency, and perhaps even the security of his very career. What about the person with extremely poor vision who yearns to be a fighter pilot, or fly domestic flights for United or Delta? Without corrective surgery, and perhaps even with it, their hopes of achieving their dreams are less than zero.

And what about the would-be athlete who wants nothing less in life than to be an Olympic athlete, a star quarterback, or a diva figure skater-but who just doesn't have the physical skills needed to achieve his or her dreams? After all, professional sports requires more than just heart, drive, and desire. It requires coordination, hand-to-eye skills, visual acuity, and in many cases, very specific physical requirements. After all, it would be difficult for a 6'4", 220-pound woman to be a petite figure skater, while it would be almost impossible for a 5' 5", 120-pound man to be a defensive lineman for the New York Jets-or the next Michael Jordan!

Vision, hearing, and coordination problems. Weight, height, physical fitness. Intelligence, IQ, the money to go to a good college. Nationality, race, religion. Fear, weakness, depression. All of these, and the list goes on and on, are disabilities of some sort. Hidden though they may be, and not labeled with a specific name or definition such as cerebral palsy, they are nonetheless real and legitimate disabilities that people face on a day-to-day basis.

My best friend in college once compared me to someone that was too short to reach the top shelf in the kitchen. She said that my "shakes" and the help I needed were no different than the short person who needed help reaching the top shelf. And she was right. All of us have shortcomings that must be dealt with, just like my shakes and someone else's shortness. When this happens, a disability occurs. Plain and simple. We all have them, we all deal with them, it's a part of life. It's how we react to those disabilities, it's how we break down the barriers they present, or work our way around them, over them, or through them, that determines how big or little those disabilities are.

In today's politically correct world, so called "normal" individuals often find it difficult to speak to, approach, or interact with those of us with disabilities. Perhaps it is simply the stereotypes propagated on TV and in the movies. Perhaps it just comes down to the basic human fear of saying the wrong thing or "messing up" by doing something or acting inappropriately in the presence of someone who is disabled.

Either way, none of this behavior helps to bridge the gap

between those of us who are disabled and those of us who aren't. That is why I called this Introduction, "We are ALL disabled." Whether it is shaking or being too short to reach the top shelf in the kitchen, we are all saddled with disabilities that we need to overcome. Just think how much better we would get along if we all had this attitude of varying degrees of disability-as opposed to "us" and "them."

After all, my physical limitations do little to affect the intellectual pursuits I engage in on a daily basis, many of which my so-called "normal" friends or family find beyond their reach. So, which one of us is disabled now? Does the fact that I can reach the top shelf in the kitchen make me more or less disabled than the short guy who can't?

All disabilities present a barrier. Whether that barrier affects your career, your health, your social life, your intellectual pursuits, even your love life, it needs to be addressed. More often, it needs to be overcome. But how?

Pathways are more than just those pleasant sidewalks lining the park. They are ways around your barriers. Whether your pathway takes you straight through an obstacle, around an obstacle, or over or under it, is largely determined by your personality. There is no wrong way or right way around your own personal barriers. That's why they're called "personal."

I developed pathways around my own barriers based on my own personality. So will you. If knocking down barriers isn't your style, you'll find a way around them, or over or under them. For if you don't, the barrier wins and your disability, whatever it may be, has gotten the best of you.

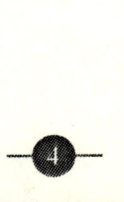

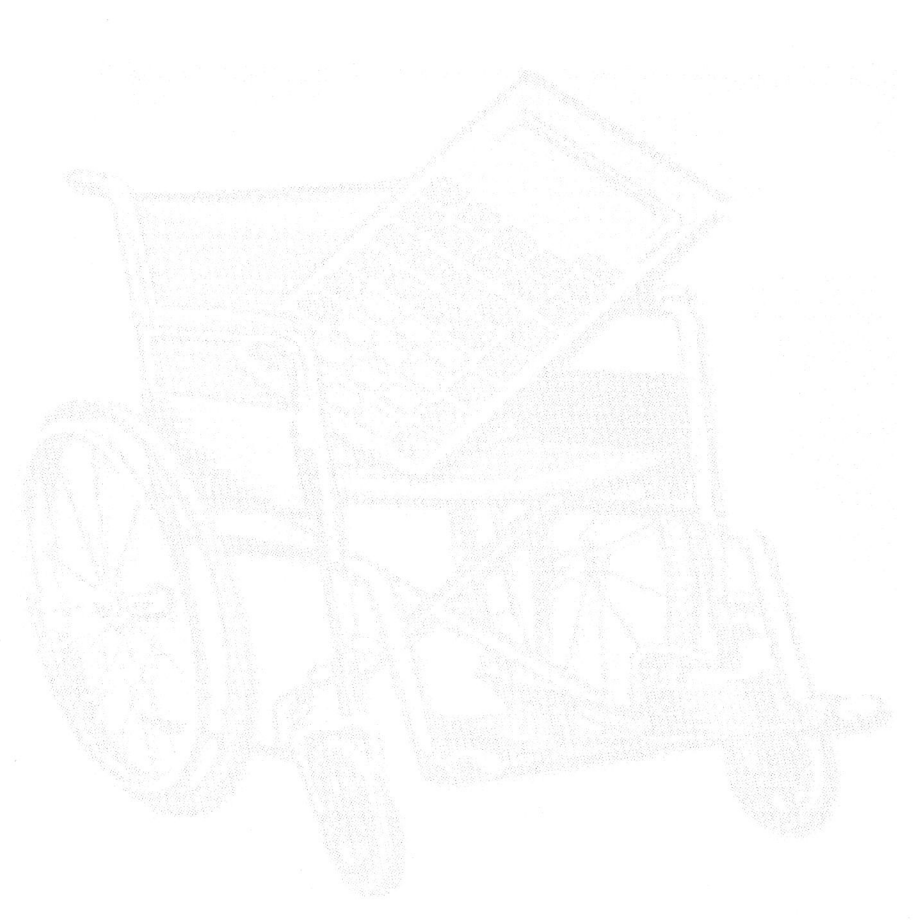

SECTION ONE:
BARRIERS IN YOUR PATH

BARRIERS IN YOUR PATH

Life is full of winding pathways-and numerous barriers popping up at the worst possible times. The rent check that's due the same week you lost your job. The radiator that begins leaking the very next week. The bad news on the other end of the phone line on the best day you've had all month. The job promotion you just missed out on, the girl that never calls back, the failing grade that should have been passing.

Success is defined by how you deal with those barriers. Do you avoid them altogether and run away? Do you forge ahead, breaking them down, squeezing around them, or leaping over them in a single bound?

While we can't all be Superman or Superwoman, it's nice to break down a few barriers now and then. Whether they be at work or at home, in school or in love, barriers do often arise-and they do need to be overcome.

But how? How do you get that job promotion? How do you score that passing grade? How do you keep moving forward when your every waking instinct is to pull up the covers, snuggle deep inside, and simply go back to bed?

Admittedly, it's not easy. Especially when you have a disability. How much harder is it to pay that rent check-when you can't even write? How much harder is it to get from Point A to Point B-in a wheelchair? How are you supposed to get your message across-when 5 out of 10 people can't even understand what you're saying?

These and many other disabilities make modern life all the more challenging-and modern barriers all the more unique. For that reason, it is more important than ever to face those barriers with courage, foresight, ingenuity, and passion.

In the following stories, I'll show you how . . .

BARRIERS PLACED BY OTHERS

ENVISION THE POSSIBILITIES

Hope comes from within. So never let someone else put a damper on your dreams, no matter who they are . . .

Who knows what makes someone want to be an accountant? Is it the neat pile of toys in their crib? The calculators and abacuses and legal pads requested in their yearly letters to Santa? Perhaps it's that very first word problem in math class and the triumph they feel when they finally solve it-long before the rest of the class!

Either way, I was bitten by the "accountant bug" as early as high school, and so naturally wanted to take the introductory accounting class offered at my high school. After all, it made perfect sense to me: I wanted to be an accountant, there was an accounting class, and I would take it. Period. End of story.

But as has happened so often in my life, a barrier that shouldn't have been there was soon placed in my pathway to becoming an accountant. And it didn't come from myself, or my fellow students, or the principal, or my family or anyone else, for that matter. It came from the very people who were supposed to be nurturing my education and encouraging me to learn all that I could: My teachers!

Both my Special Education teacher *and* the high school accounting teacher were dead-set against me taking the accounting class, which made such perfect sense to me. Their reason may have seemed perfectly reasonable to them at the time, but would prove quite ironic some eight years later.

For starters, they thought the class full of lengthy formulas and delicate equations would move too fast for someone with a disability. Why CP would limit my thought processes, they could not explain. But the fact remained that instead of telling me "you can," they told me "you can't."

To add insult to injury, both teachers firmly agreed that not only would the class be too fast-paced for *me*, but that I would slow the rest of the class down!

So why is this story so ironic?

Not only would I go on to graduate from one of the nation's finest colleges, with the top accounting program in the nation, but I would eventually obtain that thing which I had pursued so faithfully since high school eight years earlier: I would pass my CPA exam!

Like so many other people, the two teachers in this story saw my disability and instantly thought of what I "couldn't" do, instead of what I *could* do.

Had I listened to them, I would have actually believed that accounting class was too fast-paced for me and that I would slow the rest of the class down. Had I listened to them, I might have even given up my dream of becoming an accountant right there, on the spot. But then, where would I be now?

And while I had many wonderful teachers cross my pathway during my school experience, not to mention afterward, these two were certainly not among that number. We all know that students are supposed to listen to their teachers, especially when two of them are so equally in agreement.

But had I listened to those two teachers, and actually believed what they were telling me that I *couldn't* do, I firmly believe that I would not be where I am today. They were not alone, of course. Many people along the pathways of my life have tried to tell me what I couldn't do, but luckily, just as many have told me what I *can* do. Not the least of whom is myself!

THE LESSON

The lesson here is not to defy your teachers. It is also not that all teachers are bad. The lesson is not to go into accounting, or to do the opposite of what your teachers say, or even to prove whoever you can wrong, whenever you can. The lesson is a more private one. A more internal one: Listen to your heart and always, always, *always* envision the possibilities in your life.

So many family members, teachers, and even strangers will tell you, "That's impossible!" Who knows? Maybe they are just doing it to be nice. I honestly don't believe that the two teachers in this story were out to get me or trying to be spiteful just for spite's sake. In fact, looking back, I doubt they even thought they were doing anything wrong at all.

In their eyes, I was disabled. That equaled many things in their minds, I'm sure. One of those things, obviously, was that I was "slow." Perhaps they are right, in some ways. I can't run a 4-minute mile or leap over tall buildings in a single bound. But at least give me the chance. Don't crush a dream before it even has the chance to become a reality.

In your own life, I imagine you've come across the same type of people. People who think they are doing you a favor by not letting you fall on your face or trip over your own shoelaces. But I think disabled people hear "you can't" more than enough in their lifetimes.

I don't think anyone needs to add to that, let alone your teachers. But no doubt about it, they will. Whether they are trying to do what's best for you, or just trying to make *their* lives easier, you will undoubtedly come across the same kinds of teachers, or bosses, or social workers, or other people in your life.

They will talk. You will listen. But my advice is this: Don't dwell on the impossible; *envision* the possible instead. I knew I wanted to be an accountant, and I knew I could take that class, and pass it with flying colors. In the end, I passed something more important: My CPA exam.

Not because I listened to two well-meaning teachers. But because I listened to myself. I hope you will always do the same.

JOURNAL ENTRY:

Can you remember a time when someone told you what you could or couldn't do? Write about how that made you feel, and tell about how you overcame **their** limitations for yourself.

WORKING WITH THE SYSTEM

*From school boards to state disability laws, many of us are often in contact with local and county officials. But I've found that working **with** the system is the best way to "beat" the system . . .*

When I was in 6th grade I was completely mainstreamed, taking 100% regular education classes just like the rest of the kids. While I thought I was doing just fine, my 6th grade teacher was apparently having a tough time dealing with me. In fact, she felt like I was slowing the entire class down.

And so, when it came time for my annual Individual Education Program, or IEP, to be filled out and signed, my teacher highly-recommended me. For a self-contained Special Ed classroom, that is!

While it equaled a death sentence for me, this teacher was only trying to help: She thought that that way I could be in a classroom with students who were progressing at the same rate I was.

Fortunately, my mother had gone to college for, of all things, a Special Education degree. Her years of experience and training were soon about to pay off-in spades-for my future. Mom knew that the 6th grade teacher's decision to move me back from a mainstream classroom to a self-contained Special Ed classroom was not just a simple decision, but a pivotal point in my public school career.

For starters, the timing was crucial. Going from mainstreamed classrooms back to the Special Ed department in 7th grade, the very beginning of my junior high school career, would label me unfairly. It would also limit the electives and extra classes I had so been looking forward to at the middle school. Leaving elementary school was supposed to be a new beginning, not a death sentence!

Secondly, the hopes and dreams that I had for myself, the goals and plans, the advanced degrees and professional occupation I envisioned could only be obtained through competing on a level playing field with those in the mainstream population of public education. Going back into a Special Ed classroom would severely limit my options for the future. A future both myself and my family had great hopes for.

And so my Mom utilized all her teaching skills and Special Ed background to not just fight with, but *work* with, the local school board to see that my individual educational needs were being met. A decision I would be ever-thankful for.

After her initial meeting with the school board, we learned that they had two main points they were using to try to steer me back into a Special Ed classroom, points that have since become extremely ironic in light of my personal-and career-choices.

First, to allow me to remain in the mainstream student population, they wanted me to agree to one major stipulation: I could no longer talk, at all, in class. No suggestions. I couldn't answer questions-let alone ask them! Instead, my personal aid would have to ask and answer questions for me, as if I was speaking a foreign language and needed an interpreter. For once, my Mom didn't need her Special Ed degree to realize that this one was not only unfair-but unlawful as well. (And isn't it ironic that, 10 short years later, I would speak at my college graduation!)

Second, the local school board felt that by not being able to engage in outdoor activities with the other "normal" students, I would not be able to participate in-or keep up with-my fellow classmates. Yet what they failed to realize was that I had been-and would continue to be-a longtime Boy Scout. Why, I probably had twice as much "outdoor experience" as the rest of the boys in my class! (Irony #2: Upon graduating from the 8th grade, just two short years later, I would receive the Presidential Academic and Fitness awards. How's *that* for outside activity?)

After a long summer of going back and forth with a stubborn and unyielding school board, my Mom and I learned that we finally had a Due Process court date. Heading off to my yearly retreat for two weeks of Easter Seals summer camp, I looked forward to the last day, which just happened to be my court date as well.

Driving up herself, so that I could attend my own hearing, my Mom had a grim look on her face as soon as I saw her pull in to the camp entrance. When she got out of the car, my Mom said, "Rob, I have some bad news. The key person for the other side is on vacation. Can you believe that?"

Naturally, the Due Process hearing was delayed. In fact, it was never even held. On the first day of junior high school, I was indeed allowed to attend regular classes with the mainstream student body. Apparently, our arguments had finally won them over. Also, I learned that, additionally, the school board would pay for the services of a typing teacher for me.

Though I was entering 7th grade, I still had no formal writing skills because of my disability. It was felt that typing would be one way for me to have a form of written communication so that I could turn in my own papers and assignments. So not only had we won the right for me to be in the mainstream community, but I had the bonus of learning how to type as well!

THE LESSON

While I do regret the fact that I had to endure the ups and downs and legal wranglings of a formal Due Process hearing, I am nonetheless grateful for the experience-and the lesson it taught me. Thanks to my Mom's Special Ed experience, not to mention her maternal guidance, I learned that sometimes working *with* the system is the best way to "beat" the system.

We could have fought tooth and nail on every count, could have gone to the newspapers right away and pled our case to the public, hired an attorney, and "fought dirty" in a hundred or more other ways. Instead, my Mom's steady hand and firm guidance taught me to believe in the system, and in the end, she - and thus "we" - prevailed.

Working with the system not only got me what I wanted, a seat back inside a mainstream classroom so that I could pursue my hopes and dreams, it got me even more: The skills and training of a qualified typing instructor, who in turn opened the door to a whole new world of written communication, formerly closed to me. Followed closely by a new typewriter and, eventually, a computer, I was finally able to put my words, thoughts, and emotions down on paper, as I'm doing "write" now.

Who knows? Had my Mom and I chosen to "fight" the system, instead of working with it, the stars might not have aligned in just the right way and I wouldn't be writing this today.

So even though you can't be with my Mom in person, at least learn from her guidance. Never let the system roll over you. Ever. But read each situation for its specific problems-and solutions-and realize that sometimes you catch more flies with honey than vinegar!

JOURNAL ENTRY:

     Discuss a time when you felt it was better to compromise than fight? Was the result as positive as you had hoped? Why or why not?

PICKING YOUR BATTLES

It's never easy to face discrimination on a day-to-day basis. But when that discrimination stands in the way of financial security, it makes it doubly hard-and totally unacceptable . . .

It was my sophomore year of college and I needed a job over the long Christmas break, *any* job. Like any other college student, I needed money. Money for my car, money for my clothes, money for my extras at the college I was attending, money for all sorts of little odds and ends that don't go away simply because you happen to be disabled.

Therefore, it was time to search the want ads for a job that would be well suited to me. While many with disabilities have neither the confidence nor the support group to enter into the modern workforce successfully, I was emboldened by my decent GPA and recent success as a college freshman. If my disability did not prevent me playing as an equal and a peer on the now level playing field of college life, it certainly wasn't going to stop me from getting a part-time job for a little gas, movie, and spending money!

Of course, life has a way of throwing up barriers your mind can rarely foresee, and before long I realized that the discrimination and prejudices I had worked so hard-and successfully managed-to overcome in school were not limited to the halls and classrooms I had recently graduated from.

In fact, they were everywhere. And I was about to come face to face with them at almost every turn I took in my fruitless job search. I could write an entire book on this subject alone, but one experience stands out in my mind and serves as a great example of what I came up against-and eventually triumphed over:

A big-name, nationally advertised department store (that would cringe if they ever heard this story) was hiring. As a successful individual possessing a sound mind and body, not to mention all of the attributes requested in the newspaper ad, I made a phone call to the department store's Human Resource department.

Although my disability affects my speech slightly, I am clearly understandable both in person *and* over the phone. I try my best to speak slowly and enunciate, if only for the benefit of my listener, and anyone paying even the slightest bit of attention to me usually has no problem understanding what I am saying. However, it was apparent right from the start that the person on the other end of the phone in Human Resources was finding it a struggle to understand me.

"Excuse me?" she said.

"What?" she kept repeating.

"Could you repeat that," was mentioned several times.

In the end, she stated flat-out that although the ad was run only that weekend, all of the holiday positions had already been filled. Dejected, I hung up and reassessed my plan. While I knew that department store jobs were much sought after and reasonably simple to perform, I also knew that they weren't going like hot cakes in the course of one single day!

And so I bided my time and waited several hours to call back, hoping that the phone would be answered by another Human Resources representative who might be more reasonable in his or her dealings with me. As expected, the first girl I talked to was on her lunch break-or on another line. Either way, a stranger picked up with a pleasant, "Human Resources department, how can I help you?"

When I announced, very slowly and understandably, that I was interested in applying for one of the positions in the paper, I again experienced another frustrating round of "What's", "Huh's", and "I can't understand you's."

Finally, I was once again told that the positions were all full and that the department store in question was no longer hiring, but "thank you for calling."

Frustrated, but not yet giving up, I asked my Mom to call that night and inquire about jobs at the very same department store, Human Resources department, and phone number. In no time, and quite pleasantly I might add, she was informed that the department store in question was indeed hiring for the holiday and to come on down and apply in person.

Naturally, I did just that. But without the aid of my trusty computer and printer, I could not fill out the application myself and the various Human Resources representatives I encountered were afraid that if I could not even fill out my own application, I would need heavy supervision and would be hard to deal with.

In the end, I lost that battle and did not, in fact, end up working for this department store. (Although the manager did eventually apologize for stereotyping me!) And while I was unaccustomed to losing battles, I realized that things *do* happen for a reason. During that Christmas break, I was able to relax and spend some much-needed time with my family-meaning that I didn't need as much money as I'd originally planned.

THE LESSON

The lesson here is a simple one: Pick your battles. Obviously I am not a quitter, or you would not be sitting here today reading this book-because there would be no book. But one thing I learned over the course of my life is that there are some battles not worth fighting, let alone *winning*.

Having a disability does not entitle me to get a job simply because of my disability. For instance, I instinctively knew that a big-name department store whose Human Resources representatives were openly discriminating against me would be severely hampered by a negative publicity campaign. And after appearing in several local newspapers by this point, I knew who and where to call to make this happen. And quickly.

But what would I have gained by putting the pressure on this department store to hire me, if only because of my disability and the recognition a well-timed newspaper story might bring to light? Management would have never forgiven me, and word would have quickly spread to my coworkers of how I got my job. They would have made my life there miserable, and I would have won the battle only to lose the war.

Instead, I saw the writing on the wall and realized that I would do well to look elsewhere, for not only my own happiness, but my own sanity as well!

So in the end, it was *I* who won, not the department store . . .

Very often, picking your battles can bring unexpected victories. Perhaps you, too, have lost one job only to find a better one. Or perhaps not getting a job you really wanted was the impetus for you going back to school or pursuing a different career path that ended up being more to your liking. Who knows, maybe getting a less desirable job even put you directly in the path of a future spouse!

The modern world is full of fierce battles-occupational, personal, and spiritual. I learned that being disabled does not exclude me from those battles. Nor should it you, whether you are disabled or not. Battles will come and go. Some will be fierce struggles, others will be minor skirmishes. Either way, the battles you pick to fight will make all the difference in your happiness, success, and positivity.

JOURNAL ENTRY:

Was there ever a time in your life when you felt that the perceptions of others were getting in your way? Write about how you dealt with their perceptions, and proved them wrong:

AVOIDING PITY PARTIES

No matter how confident and positive you feel about yourself, there will never be a shortage of people having pity parties for you-whether you want them or not!

I have always been a spiritual person, and, while I don't attend church regularly, I do believe strongly in the Lord and feel that he has put me on this earth for a specific reason. Church has always calmed my nerves and filled me with the spiritual guidance I need to break through the many and varied barriers that litter my own personal pathways. But more than just support of a divine nature, I have met many friends there as well.

One such friend eventually asked me to speak at a local Presbyterian church where he was a member. Not wanting to miss this golden opportunity to motivate or inspire a captive, not to mention spiritual, audience, I gave my favorite presentation on "barriers" and "pathways," much of which can be found in this book.

When it was over, I felt that I had given a slightly more rousing performance than usual, and was further inspired when my friend opened up the floor for questions after I was through speaking.

From the back of the room, a man stood hesitantly and spoke slowly, as if giving a confession: "Rob," he admitted honestly, "Before the speech began, I felt pity for you. But now that the speech is over, I really respect you for all that you've done in your life. Can you ever forgive me for the way I felt?"

You could have heard a pin drop in that room as the entire audience awaited my answer. After much thought and careful consideration, however, I replied quite honestly, "No, I don't forgive you."

But I had a valid reason for refusing this man's simple request. After all, he had been programmed by society to pity me- and people just like me. Movies, books, family, friends, TV, commercials, all portray those with disabilities as poor unfortunates who need to be helped.

Yet I could tell from this man's enlightened statement that he obviously didn't feel pity for me himself. In his true heart of hearts, he obviously saw me as just another human being like everyone else in that room. So to forgive him would be to admit that he'd done something wrong in the first place.

To forgive him would acknowledge that he'd been *guilty* of something . . .

Yet by not forgiving him, I was sending him, and the rest of the audience as well, a clear message that he was guilty of nothing more than misinformation, brought to him by none other than a society who was too worried about being *politically* correct to be *morally* correct.

I didn't think it was fair to forgive a man for something he hadn't really done on his own. I felt the better course of action would be to point out what society had done to him, but more importantly, what I had been able to do for myself-in spite of a society who often pitied me.

That was the best answer I could give him, and much more powerful, I thought, than mere forgiveness . . .

THE LESSON

The story above has most likely happened to all of us at one point or another, though maybe not so pleasantly-or spiritually. For "pity" is an ugly word, and an even uglier emotion. And one few disabled people, if any, look forward to being on the receiving end of.

No matter how often we are . . .

I know that some people in that room were probably quite surprised by my strong reaction to this man's confession. In fact, I'm sure some were even offended. After all, here was this poor man braving the harsh reaction of the crowd to stand up and bear his soul to the rest of us. How dare I refuse to forgive him?

But hadn't I just stood up to bear my *own* soul to the very same crowd? Hadn't I risked more than this man to share my *own* story with people, time and time again? And who was I to forgive him anyway? Just because I was disabled didn't make me the authority on ALL disabled people.

How many times has this happened to you? How do you handle pity? Would you have reacted differently in the same situation? Or maybe you already have?

All I can do in life is act on my own instincts. My instinct in this particular situation told me that this man was having a real breakthrough in his understanding of disabilities, and my forgiveness would have severely limited his progress in this all-important matter.

I think we owe it to ourselves, and to each other, to face pity head on and confront it on a case by case basis. It is hard enough to find equality in a world that looks down on the disabled, why contribute to that by forgiving those who feel pity for us?

Look into your hearts and ask yourself, "Do I deserve pity?"

If, and when, you find that the answer is "no," this lesson will be all the more easy to implement in your own life.

JOURNAL ENTRY:

Discuss what pity means to you. Now write about a time when you came up against pity face to face. How did that make you feel? What did you do about it? What might you do differently about it now?

BARRIERS PLACED BY YOURSELF

QUITTING IS NOT AN OPTION!

For a frisky six-year old, Daycare is a place of wonder and amazement, where many lessons are learned. But sometimes, life's biggest lessons come from within . . .

I was about six-years-old when I was taught one of the most valuable lessons anyone with-or without-a disability could learn. It was a normal day, although now the lesson itself stands out more than the weather, or what I had for snack-time, or even the clothes I was wearing.

I do remember the grassy green of a playground, however, and the rousing game of soccer being played by a handful of the other children and myself. No doubt designed by the crafty Daycare staff as an effective way of wearing us all out before nap time, what was merely a game of friendly soccer for the rest of the kids suddenly became for me a test of wills.

Like so many other physical activities the so-called "normal" kids gave neither worry nor heed to, I had to play twice, if not three or four times, as hard just to keep up. When I needed my hands NOW, they nonetheless got there when they were good and ready! When I needed my legs to go HERE, they occasionally went THERE!

Meanwhile, a field full of frisky, would-be soccer stars passed me by like speeding traffic zips by a skateboarder, making me feel, as was so often the case in my childhood, small and insignificant. Who knows why this soccer game out of all the other soccer, kickball, tether ball, or other games drove me over the edge. Who knows why the other children's taunting and giggles affected me on this day more than on many others. Who knows why a disability I had learned to live with for six long years now should suddenly cause me so much grief.

All I know is that I didn't *know* - I just reacted. After missing yet another goal or flubbing yet another pass, I gave up. Perhaps all the years of being different suddenly caught up with me, as they sometimes will. Perhaps I had been called one too many a name, been the object of one too many a whisper. Perhaps I was just good and tired of not being like everybody else. Who knows, perhaps I was just good and tired of being good and tired!

Whatever the reason, I quit playing soccer and walked off the field. For the first time in as long as I could remember, perhaps even for the first time *ever* - I quit! Let the other kids kick some stupid ball around a half-pint soccer field, I was through. Done for. Kaput.

Later that evening, as my father came to pick me up, I watched in silence as he and the Daycare supervisor spoke in hushed tones. I could tell from the disappointed look on his face that she was relating the soccer story, and I wondered why. After all, a hundred different kids a day did stupid stuff, from spilling paint to drooling on themselves to spilling juice. Why was one lousy kid quitting one lousy soccer game important enough to tell my father about?

When I look back upon that day now I realize that the well-meaning Daycare worker had obviously been concerned about my frustration - and my uncertain future. I'm sure, sensing my disappointment in myself, she only wanted my father to do something to make sure that I wouldn't quit anything again, even something so small as a soccer game.

After all, if you quit the small stuff, what's gonna happen when you run into the big stuff?

My father, it seems, would not disappoint her. All the way home, he seethed with untold anger. A gruff man already, his silence and actions grew more tense by the moment. Finally, just before reaching home, my father turned to me and spoke the words I would never, ever forget: "Once you begin something, you never, ever quit. In this family, quitting is *not* an option!"

And that was it. So endeth the lesson. Since that day, whether it's a scratch soccer game or graduating from one of the country's best colleges, I've heeded that advice: For me, quitting is definitely NOT an option!

THE LESSON

The lesson my father taught me that day so many years ago was a simple one: "Once you begin something, you never, ever quit. In this family, quitting is not an option!"

The words were simple, almost sparse. Nothing that didn't need to be said was uttered. No wasted energy, no big words. No roundabout Biblical story of heroes and heroines who prevailed against big odds. No "win one for the Gipper" speeches for *my* Dad. He knew that I would heed his words, because for me, they would mean the difference between success and failure; the difference between ultimate survival and a miserable life full of repeated failures and deep depression.

My father knew that for me, especially, quitting would only lead to a lifetime of disappointment and regret. While thousands, if not millions, of kids had walked off of a soccer field in their day without notice or comment, I was special. And special in a good way, as my family and friends were quick to point out.

While no one could blame me for slowing down, wimping out, or giving up, no one I knew could quite abide by it either. And neither should you . . .

Whether your are disabled or not, young or old, tall or short, black or white, "QUIT" is spelled with the same four letters. (And you know what they say about 4-letter words!)

If something is worth doing, it's worth doing right. If something is worth beginning, it's worth seeing through to the end. Whether it is a personal relationship, a class, a degree, a private matter, or a business venture, it behooves you to see it through to the end.

Celebrities, sports stars, CEOs, Olympic athletes and other heroes and heroines are not simply "lucky" people born with silver spoons in their mouths. They are dedicated people who realized a goal early on and stuck to it through thick or thin. While their lives may seem glamorous and easy, none of us were ever there for the hard times.

For the times when the power was shut off or the phone calls went unanswered. For the struggles and the challenges and the obstacles set in their pathways. Through blood, sweat, and tears these people battled their demons and stuck to their cause.

Whatever else has been said about you, know that this much is true: There has never been a person like you-ever. And there never will be again. Your history is unwritten, and you are its only author.

So, what type of book will you write for yourself? And how will you ever know, if you don't see it through to the end?

JOURNAL ENTRY:

Was there ever a time in your life when you felt like giving up? Write about that time, and about the event-or person-who helped you stay on your very own pathway of life?

YOUR DISABILITY IS NOT AN EXCUSE

Having a disability is no picnic. Likewise, it is no excuse for failing to do those things that you can (and should) do for yourself . . .

I always loved it when my grandmother came to visit me. She was sweet and gentle and kind and, if the truth be told, she always made life in my house just a little bit easier.

After all, my parents were definitely of the "he can do it himself" school of thinking. Be it finishing my own homework or applying to a college of my own choosing, both of my parents stressed independence every step of the way.

I don't know if it was tough love or just the knowledge that life would be harder later on if I didn't stand on my own two feet right *now*, but my parents were ever-vigilant about seeing that I did as much for myself as I possibly could. And that included making my own lunch!

But one time, however, a simple sandwich taught me a lesson I wouldn't soon forget:

I was 11- or 12-years-old at the time. Old enough indeed to be making my own lunch. And as my grandmother was due for a lunch-time visit, my wise father made it quite clear that I was to make my own sandwich before she got there, and not simply wait for her to arrive and have her do it for me.

Still, I was wise in my own ways, and getting people to do things for me had become one of them. Claiming that I wasn't hungry "just yet," I indeed waited for my grandmother to arrive and, after the dust had settled and my parents were out of earshot, I asked my dear old grandmother to fix me a sandwich.

Well, as luck (or family gossip) would have it, my father soon found out about my sneaky tactics and was, in a word, furious! Not only had I directly disobeyed one of his orders, but as he saw it, I had thrown in the towel instead of finishing the fight.

Even though the task was putting together a simple lunch-time sandwich, the lesson was the same: "Don't ever use your disability as an excuse," he thundered. "Don't use it as a crutch."

"But I wasn't," I countered. "I just wasn't hungry when you told me to make a sandwich, but I was later."

But Dad wasn't buying it. "No you weren't," he replied, catching me in another lie. "You were playing the poor, little handicapped boy and I will not stand for that. First someone makes you a sandwich, but from there it snowballs. Next, someone is finishing your homework for you. From there, someone is taking your tests for you. Or taking your notes. Where will it end?

"The fact is, if you can do something for yourself, you should. Don't use your disability as an excuse, and don't ever let me catch you playing 'poor little handicapped boy' again. I won't stand for it. And you shouldn't either."

Of course, my Dad was right. I *was* playing the poor little handicapped boy, and we both knew it. Using my grandmother to fix me a sandwich was the lazy way out, and if my parents hadn't been so adamant about doing things for myself, I might never have made it this far.

Might, nothing. I KNOW I wouldn't have made it this far.

THE LESSON

The lesson my father, and by extension, my grandmother, taught me that day so many years ago was a simple one: Your disability is not an excuse!

It's not an excuse for failure. It's not an excuse for giving up. It's not an excuse for taking the easy way out. It's not an excuse for acting cute. It's not an excuse for whining or complaining or wimping out.

These things may happen. They've happened to me. They've happened to my friends. Chances are, they've happened to you and *your* friends as well. Fear and anger and disappointment and guilt are all human emotions, so why should those of us with disabilities be immune to them?

However, success and ambition and dreams and desires and goals are likewise human emotions that are universal despite race, nationality, religion, or creed. Why should those with disabilities be immune to these emotions as well?

The fact is, we are not. We are just like everybody else and that means that what we can do for ourselves, we should. I'm not saying to move mountains or knock yourself out trying to bench press 300 pounds. (Unless you really, really want to!) What I am saying is not to use your disability as an excuse or a "crutch" in order to get out of doing something that you're perfectly capable of doing for yourself.

We all get tired. We all get sore. We all get bruised and battered and defeated and depressed. But the "we" in this case is the entire human race, and not just those of us who are disabled. To play on an equal playing field with the rest of humanity, we must do as much as we can for ourselves. We all know our strengths, we all know our weaknesses. Most importantly, we all know our limitations.

But aside from our limitations, the rest of the world is our oyster and there's no reason we shouldn't suck the life out of, well, life. Letting my grandmother make my sandwich that day so long ago was a little thing. Let's face it. Grandmothers make sandwiches for their grandchildren every day of the year.

But my father was right when he told me not to play the "poor little handicapped boy." Which, of course, was exactly what I was doing. It was easier that way. Quicker. Faster. But as they say, nothing worth doing well is worth rushing, and those of us with disabilities know that most things just take a little longer.

So don't rush. Don't give up. And don't let others do for you those things you know certainly well that you can do for yourself. And I won't either . . .

JOURNAL ENTRY:

Was there ever a time in your life when you knew that you used your disability as a crutch-and got away with it? Explain how you felt, and how you would act differently in the same situation today.

(NOT) MAKING THE GRADE

In my personal classroom of life, getting a "D" in Calculus was just as bad as getting an "F"-in life!

Throughout grade school, middle school, and high school, my strongest subject-by far-was mathematics. The figures and formulas, diagrams and theorems, while confusing and befuddling many of my classmates, only challenged me to understand them more fully, which paid off in continually strong grades throughout my public schooling.

So when I entered the University of Illinois as a freshman in the fall of 1991, I decided to plunge into my very first math class headfirst. It was Calculus. Unfortunately, the teacher was not very good. But I had run up against that problem in my schooling before, and had learned long ago that you only get *out* of a class what you put *into* it, no matter how good-or bad-a teacher you have.

As the semester wore on, I began to find Calculus more and more difficult. I was discovering what so many of my fellow freshman were already learning: College wasn't quite as easy as high school! Yet, somehow, I just hadn't switched gears yet. Halfway through the semester, I discovered that I was receiving a failing grade in my Calculus class. I wasn't exactly shocked, but the disastrous grade did make me face up to the reality that if I didn't get a handle on this class-and soon-I was going to fail it for real.

At that point, I got a tutor to help me several evenings a week. This step turned out to be a double-edged sword. On one hand, I flourished with my tutor. His explanations of the complicated formulas and symbols seemed to make perfect sense-at the time. Unfortunately, it was only when I returned to class that the two versions of the same problem had me even more confused than before!

By the time the class was finally over and I received my grades, I ended up with a "D" in Calculus. The grade was doubly disappointing to me. Not only was it a lackluster way to begin my college career, but since I had always been so good at math, it was truly troubling to have such a dark blot on my otherwise stellar history.

Of course, when my Dad found out about the "D," he was furious! It would have been one thing had I *not* hired a tutor to help me, but to have two teachers working my way through one class truly revealed to my Dad that I wasn't trying my hardest.

More than just the "D," however, my father warned that college would only get harder from here on in. If I were already getting close to failing grades now, what could I expect when things *really* got rough? (As would happen so often in our relationship, I had a feeling that college wasn't the only thing my Dad was referring to . . .)

As a result of my grade-and Dad's speech-I was once again able to turn things around. The very next semester, I had the best GPA of my entire college career: 4.33 out of 5. I guess, sometimes, you've got to go down to come back up . . .

THE LESSON

Looking back upon the experience, I now realize that getting a "D" in Calculus was not the end of the world. But as my Dad was trying to impress upon me with his not-so-subtle symbolism, had I simply accepted that grade and not worked all the harder the next semester, I might not be where I am today.

I didn't just get a "D" in Calculus, after all. I had truly received a "D" in life. Despite what I thought was hard work and effort, I quickly realized that I wasn't working quite as hard or making quite so big an effort as I thought.

Blaming the teacher for being bad, blaming the tutor for confusing me, blaming my dad for not understanding, they were all designed to take the blame off of the one person most responsible for my grade: Me!

Obviously, I was not math-deficient. All through school, and even today, I excelled at math. It wasn't the teacher. I'd had bad teachers before, I've had them since, and most likely, should I decide to further my formal education at some point, I'll have them again. It wasn't the tutor. He was only trying to help. As was my father.

No, I had no one to blame but myself for that grade. And perhaps that was the most important lesson I could have learned. For relying on myself, in both the good and the bad times, is vital to my success, not just as a disabled person, but as a person in general.

Likewise, it's important for you to rely on yourself as well. Take your classes. Get a tutor. Study hard. Burn the midnight oil. In class. At your job. In life. But never forget that the buck starts-and stops-with you. Not your boss. Not your principal. Not your teacher or your tutor or your parents.

Relying on yourself to achieve, or fail, is the first step to true independence . . .

JOURNAL ENTRY:

Discuss a time when your performance was less than stellar, be it in school, at work, or elsewhere. What was the "spark" that got you back on track-and why?

YOUR ATTITUDE DETERMINES YOUR ALTITUDE

*The trouble with being an inspiration to others is-what happens when **you're** the one who needs a little inspiration yourself?*

It is hard to admit defeat. Especially after knocking down so many of the barriers I have faced in my life, and doing so in front of a loyal support group of family and friends-and even strangers-who often look to *me* for inspiration. But that is just what happened recently when several events in my life led me to make one of the most important decisions - and breakthroughs - I have ever experienced.

It started with mounting financial pressures. My credit card bills were slowly becoming unmanageable and without acquiring an extra source of income, I saw no hope of paying them off anytime in the near-or even distant-future.

On top of that, pressures at work were swiftly mounting, sending me into an all-too-familiar routine of worry and stress, stress and worry. I could barely sleep because of the worry, and lack of sleep only caused twice as much stress!

Day after day, week after week, the bills-and the pressure-mounted. I withdrew into a bleak world of pain and depression, and soon found myself in almost hopeless despair. Despite all of my successes, despite the battles I had waged and won, the inner battles raging in my very own mind were quickly getting the better of me.

Today seemed miserable, tomorrow offered little hope of anything different, and the immediate future seemed nothing short of hopeless. Fearing that I might do something serious to myself, I made the decision to seek professional help and signed myself into a local facility for mental care.

It was a grim day, but at least I had made a decision that could possibly help my present situation. And that was better than nothing. I was poked and prodded, consulted and examined, and in the quiet, reflective moments in between, I was able to observe my fellow patients.

I soon realized that what I was experiencing in my own life was nothing compared to the severe and chronic mental problems facing my neighbors and roommates. Being depressed or over-stressed was one thing, but being delusional, psychotic, or even catatonic was quite another.

Unlike my fellow patients, I realized several things about myself that first day of care: I realized that I had a loyal support group of family and friends. I realized that I was strong and free of mental disease. I realized that I was smart enough to work my way out of my present financial crisis. I realized that I didn't need shock treatment for the mild case of the blues that had combined with a bleak financial picture to bring me here.

But most of all, I realized two important things: #1: I did NOT belong here. #2: While I was not a religious man, I believed that God had put me on this earth for a purpose. And that purpose was not to sit around feeling sorry for myself. That purpose was to inform the world that I was no different from anyone else, and that CP was not something to be dreaded, feared, or ashamed of.

Where I had entered the treatment facility hopeless and depressed, I was now full of hope and desire: To share my story with others. To speak to both the disabled and the "normal." To share my message that we are all alike, despite the color of our skin, the patterns of our speech, or the shaking in our hands. And, most of all, to write this book. While all of these ideas had been playing on my mind for months, if not years, my visit to the hospital solidified them from mere dreams to a hopeful reality.

And so I was eventually released from the hospital. Once and for all. I said goodbye to the doctors and the nurses. Said goodbye to my fellow patients-those who could understand what I was saying, that is. And I returned to my old life, more determined than ever not to let myself ever reach that low point again. After all, I had too much to do!

Obviously, taking a few weeks off didn't help my financial situation, either at work or with my bill collectors. In fact, I had used up all my sick time for that year and my debt was now even greater, what with the additional medical bills! But it did provide me with the distance I needed to see that I had managed to find some small sliver of hope in the depressing and even suicidal months preceding my voluntary incarceration: I may have had CP, but my current problems were unrelated.

For one of the first times in my life, the problems I was experiencing, and their possible solutions, were completely unrelated to my disability. Having CP hadn't racked up my credit card bills. That was my own fault. And mounting pressures at work were completely unrelated to my careful speech patterns or shaking hands.

Money problems were universal, and I was finally experiencing what much of the non-disabled world experienced every single day: Life as part of the rat race! Graduating from one of the country's finest schools and passing my CPA exam were dreams come true. And now I was living the dream, even if it occasionally felt like a nightmare!

And, in living the dream, I suddenly realized that I could be an inspiration to others. Not by playing basketball or running a triathlon, but by simply raising the disability bar to play on an even field with the rest of my friends, family, and coworkers. I had accomplished something special. I had accomplished something unique. And not by magic or luck or fame or fortune, but with good, solid hard work and dedication.

If I could speak to people-classrooms, college students, even business people-and share my message of triumphing over adversity and playing the hand God dealt me, I could be more than just another corporate drone losing the rat race, I could spread the word that disabilities do not equal either giving up or staying put.

This was cause for celebration, not depression. And it was high time I realized that and got on with my life. And that's exactly what I did . . .

THE LESSON

The bills did not erase themselves, of course. And the pressures at work did not go away with one wave of my magic wand. No, like most of the rest of the world, I had to put my nose to the grindstone and make some changes in my lifestyle, spending budget, and working habits.

But the lesson here is not how to pay your bills or free up your current workload. The lesson here is to view things from a different perspective when the one you currently have is both miserable and bleak.

I had high bills. I had too much stress at work. And together the two got me down in the dumps. It was as simple as that. I wasn't depressed, or suicidal, or psychotic. I was frustrated-both financially and professionally-because of an unfortunate combination of internal and external factors.

In short, I was learning how to grow up in a grown up world. Like so many of my fellow college grads who'd recently entered the workforce with little or no preparation or experience, I was facing up to a grim reality. But it was a reality that was neither unique to me, nor unavoidable. To pay off my mounting bills and ease my load at work, I would have to work harder and spend less. Period.

But before I had a chance to feel too sorry for myself, the internal drive and barometer that had seen me break through so many of life's previous barriers served me well again: I determined my *altitude* by rearranging my *attitude*.

I was my own worst enemy, and my only solution. I could quit and give it all up, playing the poor, miserable, disabled victim who had tried his best but just wasn't good enough, or I could be grateful for the fact that my current problems were actually the result of my deepest desires coming true.

After all, if I hadn't graduated college and passed my CPA exam, I wouldn't have all this pressure at work and wouldn't have even had the job to secure my credit cards - and thus my credit card *debt* - with in the first place! I was concentrating way too much on the symptoms, and ignoring the cure.

But with one single trip to the local psychiatric facility, and a quick slap in the face from the harsh hand of reality, I soon realized that what was once a problem was now an opportunity: I had the job, the college degree, the driver's license, and all the other tools of the trade to be a normal, fully-functioning, grown up adult.

It was time to start enjoying my success, rather than fearing it . . .

It was time to stop dreading my life, and living it . . .
It was time to stop privately celebrating my joys and triumphs, but to share them with others just like myself . . .
It was time to answer the call.

How about you? What is your personal call to arms? What are your dreams and desires? What things do you want to accomplish with your life?

And what is holding you back? Is it your disability - or just fear and uncertainty? Either way, what are some ways you can break down your own personal barriers and find alternate pathways around all three?

JOURNAL ENTRY:

When was there a time in your life when you needed inspiration, only to receive it from within? Write about how you can recall that time for solace when times of trouble appear now:

MAKE PLANS, NOT WISHES

Buying my first house was a dream come true for me-or anyone with a disability. But hoping and praying would never have been enough . . .

Buying a home is a lifelong dream that eludes millions of Americans-with disabilities or without. College graduates, retirees, men, women, tall, short, young, or old, few people can afford the skyrocketing prices of a single-family home these days. In fact, the dream eluded me for several years and, like a batter with 2 strikes and 3 balls, I wasn't able to buy my house until almost the final inning. But I finally bought it, and here's how:

As an accountant, money is very important to me. Not that I covet it, or keep it under my mattress, or am greedy or cheap or anything like that. I enjoy spending my hard-earned money, as much on my family and friends as I do on myself. Through my job and position, I've been able to help out several family members who have run into debt issues, or who just wanted to buy a new car or otherwise needed a loan. Among my friends and family, I am definitely known as a "soft touch."

But I've always known that owning my own home would be a dream that eluded me if I did not plan for it, and plan for it early. And so I did. Despite having several credit cards and other purchases on time, I was always careful to pay early-not late-and to avoid costly late payment fees. Not only to avoid the extra expense they incurred, but more importantly for the irreparable damage they do to one's credit.

And so, by the year 2000, I had a spotless credit report with not one single late fee on it. Of course, I also had nothing in my savings account! Not one thin dime. Still, I approached a realtor, shopped around, and finally found a condominium in a good neighborhood with one necessity I'd always had in mind: a garage. (While southerners may not appreciate this "extra room," us northerners find it quite necessary in the chilly winter months.)

I was able to finance the house with no money down, and in my budget range, because of one thing and one thing only: My sterling credit report. Had I wavered in my desire to own my own home and foolishly fudged up my credit along the way, I would never own a home.

I was quite proud of my purchase, for many reasons. One, I had stuck to my guns and made it happen. All by myself. Not a single family member or friend - except for perhaps with the moving - helped me finance my dream home. That's pretty good for a 27-year-old. *Any* 27-year-old. But for one with a disability, it's almost entirely unheard of.

But I had done it. All by myself. No inheritance. No grant money. No endowment. Just myself, my hard work, and always, always, a good, solid, financial plan.

That planning paid off, in more ways than one . . .

THE LESSON

I could never have bought my own home without proper planning. Now, if this were a simple book on real estate, THAT would be the lesson. However, the lesson here is just as simple: Don't just rely on hopes and dreams to come true, MAKE those hopes and dreams come true!

After all, if I had simply hoped and dreamed for my own house, it would have never happened. Actually, it almost didn't. Twice! In fact, I had been down the home ownership road not just once, but twice before. All to no avail . . .

In 1996, I made my first attempt to buy a house. I looked, I shopped around, I even stargazed in local neighborhoods. I even narrowed it down to one or two favorites. But when the time came to put pen to paper, it turned out that I had neither good *or* bad credit, I had NO credit. No credit, no house.

Later, in 1998, after I'd established a little more credit, I found that I had another problem: With just a little credit, and a little down payment, my mortgage would be so high each month as to be prohibitive. In other words, my debt load would have been too big. Could I have done it? Sure. But did I *want* to? No. I wanted to relax in my new home, not stress over it day and night!

And so, for two more years, I struggled and strained to make my monthly payments on time-if not early-even when it meant not putting anything into savings, or even going without. I budgeted and planned and scrimped and saved to make those monthly payments on time. As a result, I established good credit. Great credit. Even excellent credit.

In the end, that made it possible for me to buy my house . . .

So don't just wish on a star, bank on it! Don't just make wishes, make plans. They may not be as whimsical or romantic - and they're not very fun - but they work. Look at me, I'm living proof . . .

JOURNAL ENTRY:

Has there ever been a milestone you planned and saved for? Has there ever been a hope or dream you couldn't make come true? Describe the difference between the two.

SECTION TWO:
UNDERSTANDING THE PATH

UNDERSTANDING THE PATH

As the old saying goes, there's a big difference between "walking the path, and *knowing* the path." In this case, the long, winding path we all must walk is the big one called "Life." So to know the path is to understand life itself. But understanding the path raises a multitude of additional questions in and of itself:

In particular, who will you meet along this pathway called life? Friends? Acquaintances? Enemies? People with your best interests at heart - or *theirs*? People who want to help-or hurt?

The path is full of all of the above, and many, many more. Getting along with other people as you wind your way through life is one of the hardest lessons-not to mention the most valuable - to learn. Bosses. Coworkers. Spouses. Teachers. Students. Neighbors. Family. Friends.

These are the people who can help you become a better person, and vice versa. These are the folks you spend your days- and often your nights-with. Day in, day out. Week in, week out. For months. For years. Their effect upon you - and your life - may be positive or negative. But for better or worse, you and the people you meet make up a big part of your pathway called life.

There is one more person you must deal with on this pathway: yourself. How often do we really get to know ourselves? How often do we understand our own innermost thoughts, feelings, fears, worries, hopes, dreams, and concerns?

Often, getting to know ourselves can be just as challenging as getting to know all those other people we come in contact with along the journeys our pathways bring us down. The following stories are intended to help us grow closer to each other-as well as ourselves.

UNDERSTANDING OTHERS

ACCENTUATE THE POSITIVE

Life is full of compromises. Some work in our favor, some don't-depending on whether or not you "accentuate the positive" instead of the negative.

Throughout my senior year of high school, it became more and more important to me to speak to my fellow classmates at graduation. I had worked so hard and fought so many battles during my last four years of public schooling, that I felt compelled to share my experiences-both good and bad-with my fellow graduating class. From pipe dream to reality, I found myself not just envisioning myself speaking before my fellow graduates, but mentally rehearsing the actual words I would say to them in my head. First as sentences, then as paragraphs, then as sound bites in my own mental "instant replay."

As the time to graduate drew near, I realized that I was not alone in my speaking ambitions. When it came time to apply for those coveted speaking spots, I learned that I was in company with 6 or 7 other graduates who also wanted to share their experiences with their graduating class.

Not surprisingly, our principal quickly realized that 6 and possibly 7 speakers at graduation would be just a few too many. Democratically, he invited all of the applicants into his office to discuss alternatives for a more realistic approach. It was up to all those in attendance to make a final decision about the number of graduating speakers.

Amazingly, this select group of mature soon-to-be graduates came up with a unique solution: The 4 valedictorians would be allowed to actually speak to the graduating class at our formal ceremony. Another student would give his graduation speech at the traditional senior lunch. And myself and another graduating senior would be able to write down our speech into essay form and find it printed in the formal program handed out to each and every one of our graduating classmates. While it was a bittersweet pathway around a considerable barrier, it was one that I soon grew comfortable with.

A similar experience occurred as my graduation from the University of Illinois approached. However, a compromise in this arena was met on an entirely different level. For starters, this time I had little competition for speaking to my graduating class. When I went to apply, only one other student had applied for the same coveted honor. And, since the U of I Business school split its graduation into two parts: Economics and Accounting grads at one time, Marketing and Administration at another, we were both allowed to speak.

But this time, the content of my speech was at issue, and not whether or not I would speak in the first place. After reading my proposed speech, The Dean of the Business College wanted me to come in and talk to him. It turns out that he felt my original draft of the speech was too negative. He felt that a graduating speech should be more positive and uplifting.

At first, I was disappointed by this apparent censorship. However, as I began to revise the more positive speech that I would eventually present to my graduating class, I formed the basis for this book as I began to write, perhaps for the first time, about the pathways we are presented with, the barriers we face, and how we choose to deal with them.

In essence, my initial "compromise" became a rough draft for this very book!

THE LESSON

Compromise. To some it can be a dirty word, although it's spelled with considerably more than four letters! For me, however, I have finally learned how to accentuate the positive. So can you.

For instance, in the first story, I could have been really disappointed that I wouldn't actually be presenting my speech out loud, in front of my graduating class like the four valedictorians did, or even live and in person in front of them at the only slightly less hallowed senior lunch. I could have refused to bend, and not been allowed to voice my opinions at all. I could have protested, blown up, or even boycotted the graduation!

But where would that have gotten me? In the end, after much reflection on this experience, I've come to realize that out of all 7 of those speeches, mine had the most potential to be remembered, or at least recycled, out of them all. After all, there it was, printed for posterity, published, technically, in the actual graduation program.

I've still got mine. Chances are, most of the rest of the graduating class still has theirs. While the valedictorian's speeches were heard, appreciated, and fondly recalled, mine lives on in posterity. Every reunion, every anniversary, there it is, readily printed in black and white and available for any and all to read, until the end of time.

And my second experience with speaking to a graduating class, at college no less, was even more fulfilling. Not only did I actually get to speak, live and in person, but I was given valuable editorial advice from none other than the esteemed Dean of the University of Illinois College of Business!

It doesn't get much better than that. But wait, it does! Not only did he help me realize that my speech needed a different tone, but in the rewriting of that speech I began the germ for my philosophy on handling the many and various barriers that pop up along life's pathways with one of the most important traits of all: Positivity!

Talk about ending on a "positive" note!

JOURNAL ENTRY:

When was the last time you had to compromise on something that was truly important to you? How did you handle it? How would you handle it now? Could it have ended up more positively for you in some way? Describe how . . .

ADAPTING BEFORE IT WAS MANDATED

Standing up for your rights often means making compromises to achieve the goal you have set out for yourself. Sometimes, standing up for your rights even means-sitting down!

When I was in 5th grade I didn't know much about marching band, except for the fact that I would probably never be in one! After all, "marching" anywhere wasn't one of my strong points, let alone walking in line carrying an instrument almost as heavy as myself! All that changed, however, when a forward thinking and brave man named Mark Victor approached me about one day being in the high school marching band. Although we both realized that I would never be John Philips Souza, it inspired me to knock down another barrier and make history by becoming the first disabled person ever to join the marching band at my high school-and I dare say one of the few to do so ever.

But more than that, I was impressed with Mr. Victor's forward thinking-not to mention his foresight. After all, this was only 5th grade. I had another three years yet before I'd even be eligible to march with the high school band. Yet there was Mr. Victor, already gunning his engines and putting his mind to work for how we could best ease the transition and make my appearance on the high school football field a natural one.

His first idea, and I later learned he had also been thinking about this for some time, was to have me suit up in the full band uniform and hold my instrument while sitting in a wheelchair on the parade route.

While this option was not ideal to either of us, it was indeed one way to conquer the many barriers that faced us. It was also a strong lesson in learning to compromise. After all, sitting was far from marching, by anyone's standards, let alone the high ones I was so accustomed to setting for myself. Still, it was a means to an end, and would be the least obtrusive manner in which to finagle my way onto the same playing field as the rest of the band members.

The thing that struck me the most about these marching band developments, however, was that Mr. Victor had been noodling over them for years. He was already thinking through the barriers-the wheelchair, the parade route-before I even knew there was an opportunity to be in the marching band in the first place!

And this was 1987-1988, long before inclusion and when it became "politically correct" to accommodate people with disabilities. Mr. Victor had no hidden agendas, no payoff other than to see a strong-willed person such as myself achieve a goal that had previously alluded him.

I gained a lot of respect for Mr. Victor that year, but more so for myself. Once our plan was put into action and I was finally on the playing field, uniform on and instrument in hand, the other marching band members fully accepted me and wanted me to succeed. But more than that, they treated me as an equal and truly allowed me to be myself.

For no matter whether our team was the host or the visitor, I always felt at "home" marching in the band . . .

THE LESSON

Not only playing in my high school marching band, but actually being invited to play in my high school marching band by Mr. Victor himself taught me many things: Pride, accomplishment, ingenuity, compassion, and compromise.

It also taught me that you don't always have to do everything alone, and that, every once in awhile, someone else will help you think through the barriers before they even show up.

For that's exactly what Mr. Victor did. Long before he had to, long before it was politically correct, long before inclusion, long before I was even a freshman in high school, Mr. Victor was busily plotting a way for me to get on that playing field. And not just as a special attraction or sympathetic sideshow, but as an equal.

That was maybe what impressed me the most. Mr. Victor had no hidden intentions, no secret payoff, no ulterior motive. He wanted to see me succeed, at any cost, and he wanted to see me succeed as an equal. Whether that be in a wheelchair or leaning on crutches, he saw compromise as a bridge we would cross when we came to it.

Also, neither of us saw compromise as a dirty word. For what was the bigger sin: Me never trying out for the marching band in the first place? Me giving up and lying down? Me ignoring Mr. Victor's pleas to join the band in any capacity?

Or me refusing out of pride or some other vanity not to sit in a wheelchair if that was the only way I could be on that playing field? In the end, the decision was an easy one: I would march when I could, ride when I couldn't.

In the end, it was that simple . . .

But, of course, simple had nothing to do with it. Becoming a full-fledged member of the high school marching band was a triumph that was, literally, years in the making. It was a triumph that surprised me. It was a triumph that inspired me. And it was a triumph that proved to me that even when you're not ready to knock over a barrier in your path, someone else might just be willing to lead the battle cry for you!

JOURNAL ENTRY:

Has there ever been a time in your life when the obstacles you faced seemed insurmountable? Write about how you and others have broken down those barriers and proceeded along your own pathway:

DEALING WITH MISUNDERSTANDING

Being misunderstood is an unwritten side effect of having a disability. But whose job is it to educate the public?

It was supposed to be a momentous occasion: I was finally moving into my first college dorm and I was thoroughly excited. My bags were packed, my expectations were high, and it was time to start down yet another long, winding pathway to my future dreams and goals.

Before heading off to campus, my family decided to attend a large computer show at the local county fairgrounds. In the brisk fall weather, my mom, dad, sister, and I walked around the various display booths checking out the latest hi-tech gadgets and computer products. From monitors to keyboards, software to mice, the gadget gurus and techno tyrants were displaying their finest wares.

As I wandered from booth to booth, I thought of how much technology had changed my life. Unable to write by hand, first the typewriter and then the computer keyboard had literally opened up new avenues of schoolwork-and thus opportunity-for me. Not only could I now communicate through the written word, but I didn't have to rely on someone else to translate it for me.

All by myself, I could compose and write entire school assignments, including but not limited to term papers, research reports, short stories, and even speeches, as I had done for my high school graduating class' recent program. Finally, I could translate the words inside my head onto a printed piece of paper without it looking like chicken scratch, and giving some teacher or professor the wrong impression.

Sorting through piles of half-price software and the latest hi-tech accessories, I realized that the revolution technology had wrought on my life was, in fact, making the rigors of college more accessible to me. With my handwriting so affected by my disability, writing notes and trying to keep up with the rest of my assignments by hand would have been nearly, if not entirely, impossible.

Yet through the magic of technology, I could now look forward to typing my assignments on a computer and printing them out for each one of my classes. Otherwise, who knows how short my tenure in academia might have been. The recent advances in technology had given me confidence, acceptance, and more importantly, true independence.

And as I was busy congratulating myself on making so many of my own dreams come true through the magic of technology, not to mention my own hard work and sheer determination, something unusual happened: A grown man ripped a computer mouse right out of my hand!

He wasn't just any man, of course. He was the proprietor of a particular booth at the computer show. An altogether appealing booth featuring some very cool computer mice which had captured my attention only a few minutes earlier. As I stood admiring a computer mouse shaped just like a pen, I reached out to pick it up and feel if it was as functional as it was visually stunning.

Apparently, the owner of the booth thought my disability might cause me to damage the item in some manner, and so he acted as he saw fit: By snatching the offending mouse out of my very hands!

I was surprised by the man's actions, yet not shocked. After all, how many times before had ignorant people mistaken my disability for something else? For craziness or stupidity or anger or lack of coordination or something other than what it really was?

In the end it was an unpleasant, yet fitting, way to start my college career. On one hand I had come so very far. On the other, I still had so very, very far to go . . .

THE LESSON

As if having a disability isn't hard enough in itself, being misunderstood by the general public is an unpleasant side effect. Many of us with disabilities are called names, ignored, stared at, picked on, misunderstood, underestimated, or insulted on a daily basis, if for no other reason than that we are different.

The actions of that concerned computer booth owner were no different than the cashier who asks you to repeat yourself over and over again instead of simply listening more closely. Or the coach who won't let you join the team because he doesn't think you're strong enough, or coordinated enough, or athletic enough. Or the teacher who won't let you take her class because she thinks you'll slow it down. Or the admissions rep who laughs when you show up for your college orientation. Or the human resource secretary who looks around for the hidden camera when you ask for a job application.

In a hundred different ways, the ignorance of the general public can serve to make your disability a much more difficult affair than it already is. But whose job is it to educate the public? Yours? Or theirs?

While I try to do my best to educate those around me, I also have a life to lead. Goals to achieve. Barriers to knock down. And so do you. I encourage you to do your best, each and every day, to follow your own pathway and break down your own barriers-for yourself. If you are able to educate a few people without disabilities along the way, then that is a definite bonus.

But I believe that the best education we can provide as a group is to put more and more people with disabilities in positions, occupations, colleges, classrooms, and offices in which there formerly were none. The more of us there are working or going to class or riding the bus or enjoying the employee break room with people without disabilities, the less educating we'll have to do, and the more friendships, growth, and understanding we'll **ALL** enjoy.

JOURNAL ENTRY:

Discuss an event in which your disability led to a misunderstanding of your potential as a human being. How did you find a pathway around this particular barrier?

FIGHTING STEREOTYPES

Like skin color or a foreign accent, having a disability opens one up to a wide variety of stereotypes . . . and just as many misconceptions.

Anyone who knows me knows that I am a HUGE basketball fan. If it's basketball season, you can often find me glued to the TV set cheering on my favorite teams, or perhaps even at a local college or professional game here in town. And God forbid you should ask me a question in either case! Either way, I enjoy the fierce competition and consummate skill displayed by today's excellent basketball players, not to mention the warm camaraderie and fellowship of sharing a favorite team or two with a legion of other fans just like myself.

And so when I entered college, I was thrilled to finally go back to my old high school to attend my first high school basketball game as an alumnus. Naturally, I was filled with impatience and much anticipation as I waited for my sister to get ready. She was a member of the pep band, and since we were both headed to the same game, I had mistakenly promised to drive her there.

My father, another big basketball fan, would be joining us later after he wrapped up some last minute errands. Arriving at the game a little early, I bought my ticket from a smiling older woman at the bustling gate and then returned to the gymnasium lobby to await my father's arrival. Already I could hear the squeak of the basketball player's shoes on the glistening court as they took their warm-up shots, and my impatience was running high when my father finally showed up some minutes later.

Accompanying him to the ticket gate and approaching the

same cashier as I had earlier, I was shocked and somewhat embarrassed when I overheard her say to my father, and I quote (as if I could ever forget it!): "Oh, you would be so proud of your son. He did such a good job buying his *own* ticket!"

Then she turned to me and pointed to an ad in the basketball program that stated, "WHEN YOUR HIGH SCHOOL WINS, YOU WIN A FREE VIDEO RENTAL." (Bet she was disappointed when I did not jump up and down shouting, "YIPPEE!")

Not ones to let sleeping dogs lie, it must have been pure shock that allowed my father and I to get all the way around the corner before we looked at each other and questioned whether or not we had heard the woman correctly. Naturally, we spent the next several minutes debating which item of mine we should show her: My University of Illinois student ID card-or my driver's license! (Both of us thought the latter would be a great way to scare her into being that much more of a defensive driver on the road from now on!)

But in the end we merely shrugged her insulting comments off to ignorance and took our place in the crowded stands. After all, there was no way her casual put down was going to ruin my first game of the season. Still, it was hard to forget the incident and I found myself steaming-and laughing-about it long after the game had started.

Did she not realize that not only had I bought my own ticket, but that I had driven myself to the game as well? And not just driven myself, but my sister as well. How dare she assume that simply because I had a slight speech impediment and a mild case of palsy in my hands that I was somehow too "slow" to buy my own basketball ticket! Where did she get off?

And, more importantly, what could I do to prevent it from ever happening again?

THE LESSON

Prejudice. Insults. Stereotypes. They raise their heads at the most inopportune moments, don't they? There I was, all set to enjoy my first high school basketball game as a former graduate, but the not-so-innocent comments of a total stranger not only marred the experience for me, but have stayed with me ever since.

And therein lies the lesson: How you react to prejudices, insults, and stereotypes is all up to you. Logically, I knew that old woman was merely trying to be nice. She saw, through her naive or perhaps ignorant eyes, someone doing something far beyond their capabilities. As such, she saw fit to compliment me-to my father.

I am quite certain that she intended to improve our night, not ruin it. She saw an opportunity to say something "nice," and she took it, assuming incorrectly that my father would be proud. Yet little did she know that her two short sentences had quite the opposite effect.

After all, my father-and myself-had much more to be proud about than merely buying a simple basketball ticket. How about breaking the bonds of my special education classes and being successfully mainstreamed into the regular classes when everyone else thought I would get swamped? How about getting my driver's license? How about my first part-time job?

Yet what good did it do me to get mad at this woman? Was it hurting her? Nope. Just me. Yes, I was hurt. Yes, I was embarrassed. But only I had the power to let her comments hurt me, embarrass me, or defeat me. And perhaps therein lies another lesson: Do what you can to educate others, but take care of yourself first.

I could have spent hours educating that poor woman on the ups and downs of every one of my successes. But what would it have accomplished? Besides backing up the line to buy tickets, that is! No, I chose to make myself a better person instead.

No doubt you have run into this same type of well-meaning person in your life as well. Perhaps at school, perhaps at work, perhaps even at home. My advice is to fight becoming stereotyped as often as possible. With words, yes. But with actions most of all. For in the end, it is not what you say to people that counts, it is what you prove to yourself that really does!

JOURNAL ENTRY:

How do you handle it when someone has stereotyped you unfairly? Talk about ways in which you could handle yourself better, or perhaps ways in which you could help others handle it better as well.

DON'T EXPECT RESPECT-UNTIL YOU EARN IT!

Like money or trust, RESPECT must be earned. So don't expect respect-until you earn it!

Deciding to pursue my interest in public speaking at the college level was one of the most important decisions of my career, not to mention my life. While I was buoyed by my success at the high school level, speaking on the competitive college circuit was initially intimidating to me.

Like everything else at the college level, things were going to be taken up a notch. Professors were more demanding, class loads were more rigorous, classmates were busier and more complex, and I had no doubt that public speaking on the college level would be twice as difficult as it was in high school.

I was not to be disappointed:

It was a simple Monday night during my freshman year when I walked into my first college speech meeting on the University of Illinois campus. I was nervous and apprehensive, and my future teammates, and even my future coach, proved that I had every reason to be.

From the very beginning, they all let me know that they thought my disability would prove to be just too daunting for me to ever become a productive member of the U of I Speech Team. Not only were they concerned about my slight speech impediment affecting the quality of my presentations, but they had a new concern, one I hadn't even thought of: They questioned my maturity as well. As a freshman, they were concerned that I might not have the life experiences or calm collectedness to handle myself under fire-and in front of large crowds of people.

Yet despite their hesitation, I joined the team and did go on to eventually become a productive member of the University of Illinois Speech Team. I knew I had the goods. It would just take some time to prove to the rest of the team, and my coach, that I could deliver them.

Slowly, I did. It took practice, and I realized that, as many of my teammates already suspected, I had much to learn. I benefited from the seniors, and even the juniors and sophomores, on my team. But I also benefited from the wise guidance of my coach, Dave Koslowski.

Coach Koslowski watched as I competed. Week after week, he expressed not only surprise but pride at the amount of growth, poise, and maturity I managed to promote when speaking. Taking Coach Koslowski's lead, the rest of the speech team got behind me as well. Soon I was no longer an outsider, but instead valued as a competitive and contributing teammate.

While I scored points and learned volumes, I also gained something else from that exciting first year on the University of Illinois Speech Team: Respect. I learned that respect was not something simply given to you out of hand, but something you earned through long months of hard work and effort.

Slowly, that hard work and effort earned me more respect. Eventually, my teammates' respect paid off in my current part-time job of assistant Speech coach at the nearby College of Dupage!

THE LESSON

Earning respect is a valuable lesson in and of itself, and one I gladly share with you here. Don't expect respect just because you are disabled. Despite the fact that we earn people's respect each and every day, just by managing to live a normal life with so many barriers and obstacles thrown in our individual pathways, the fact remains that we are expected to compete on an even playing field with the rest of society.

For instance, I couldn't get away with being "pretty good for someone who is disabled" on the University of Illinois Speech Team. After all, this was a top-notch competing organization from one of the best schools in the country. Simply joining the team didn't make me a contributing part of it. I had to earn that right, and earn the rest of the team's respect.

I was competing against teammates without disabilities, whose speech and mobility were unhindered and who could wax poetically through their perfect diction and agile hand-eye coordination. And not only that, I was competing against other schools whose speakers almost always surpassed even those of the U of I team.

So I couldn't just be "good enough." I had to be just plain "good."

And, with the help of Coach Koslowski and the rest of the team, I managed to get that way-and stay there. It gave me great pride to rise to the occasion and overcome the rest of the team's doubts about my potential. But not as much pride as it gave me to be respected by my teammates, my coach, the audience, and even the other team's members during those exciting speech competitions.

Like I said, the respect I earned during those heady days of speech competition didn't just boost my confidence, they gave me a leg up on a career: I am now an assistant speech coach at the College of Dupage.

Likewise, learn to earn respect in your life, instead of simply expecting or assuming it as your proper due. We all fear hard work and disappointment. But only through putting in the work, and rising to the challenge, will we ever truly earn the respect of our peers.

And respect can do wonders for your confidence level. Just look at me!

JOURNAL ENTRY:

What does respect mean to you? Describe a time when you earned respect, but didn't get it. How about a time when you desired respect, without putting the time in to earn it? Of the two events, which was the most bittersweet? Why?

UNDERSTANDING YOURSELF

BE CAREFUL WHAT YOU WISH FOR . . .

When dealing with a disability, choosing the right career-for you-can often be one of the biggest decisions of your life. So be careful what you wish for . . .

When I started course work at the University of Illinois, I was determined to become a political science major. History and world events had always been a passion of mine, and to work in such a challenging and rewarding field seemed highly desirable to me-at the time.

As I began taking classes in my chosen major, however, I soon realized that actual careers in Political Science were few and far between. As the reality of the professor's warnings and statistical employment figures sank in, I soon realized that I might want to seek greener pastures elsewhere.

As anyone with a disability can tell you, independence is a top priority. Depending on others may be a necessity at times, but it's certainly not a desirable goal when choosing one's career. And if I was to gain any form of true independence as an adult, I would have to find not just my "dream job" of becoming a political scientist, but a job that actually paid the bills!

About this time, I took an elective class in Accounting. I found the work invigorating and, better yet, the prospects for an Accounting job were much more realistic than those for Political Science majors. After much thought and consideration, I decided to change my major.

Unfortunately, as so often happens, I found a barrier sitting right in the middle of my pathway to becoming an Accounting major.

For starters, I found that I couldn't change my major until I had completed 60 hours of course work. As I was still in the beginning of my sophomore year at the University of Illinois, I was obviously a few credit hours short of this requirement.

Furthermore, the University of Illinois' College of Business is one of the top business schools in the nation, and I knew that their admission requirements would be extremely demanding. As most of my class work up until this time had been focused on becoming a Political Scientist, I did not feel quite prepared for this arduous undertaking.

Yet as the title of this book implies, I knew that there had to be some alternative way around this unique and imposing barrier. Upon doing some research of other related majors, I soon realized that a degree in Economics would, in fact, qualify me to sit for the extremely difficult CPA exam, which would be my final barrier to becoming a licensed accountant.

Therefore, as soon as I had completed 60 hours of course work, I immediately changed majors from Political Science to Economics. Once there, I discovered an aptitude for such work and, through hard work and determination, eventually acquired such competency as to meet the rigorous demands of the U of I Business School, where I was finally accepted during my junior year.

THE LESSON

"Be careful what you wish for," is an old saying that still rings true today. For our purposes, I believe that this witticism means we should always be examining-and re-examining-our decisions, whether in life, love, career, clothing, automobiles, etc.

Human beings are fascinating creatures whose judgment and decision-making processes continually evolve as we learn, grow, and experience life. What we hope, desire, and dream for as children is rarely what we hope, desire, and dream for later on in life. Particularly as adults.

Priorities change with circumstance, and the desires for independence, comfort, and personal satisfaction often outweigh our childish dreams of fame, fortune, or even traveling to the moon!

When I entered college, I couldn't see myself doing anything *but* becoming a living, working Political Scientist. My entire focus revolved around this challenging career choice, and the various rewards and satisfaction it would bring to my life. It seemed a natural fit for my curiosities and interests, and no one could dissuade me from this course of action.

However, as I grew older and experienced more of life, particularly the economic side such as bills, car payments, and rent, I realized quickly that dreams and reality rarely cross paths. While my passion for political science remained strong, so did my desire for financial independence from my parents, friends, and other family members.

Therefore, I reexamined my career goals, reevaluated my needs and desires, and developed a new plan for a job that would both satisfy my curiosities and interests, while at the same time pay the bills. After that, I took the appropriate actions to complete my required course work, change majors, enroll in the appropriate school, and pass the CPA exam, all of which I managed to accomplish to my own personal-and professional-satisfaction.

So, be careful what you wish for. Not only may it come true, but by the time it does, you may just find yourself wishing for something else entirely! Learn to blend your hopes and dreams with your present reality, and don't be afraid to continually revise your daily, weekly, and monthly goals accordingly.

The real challenge is to live, grow, and work in a continually changing-and challenging-modern world. The real *triumph* is to do so on your own terms . . .

JOURNAL ENTRY:

Write about a wish you've always had. Have you achieved it yet? How many times have you revised this wish? Is it time to revise it again?

DON'T BLAME YOUR DISABILITY

I learned a lot of things at my first "real" job. One of them was to not use my disability as an excuse . . . for anything!

When I graduated from college, like any recent graduate I looked forward to getting steady employment and building a solid resume at a respectable company as I began the slow but inevitable climb up the corporate ladder.

The fact that I had a disability was, no doubt, high on the minds of those sitting across from me in every interview, but I am proud to say I didn't let it slow *me* down. I had achieved a lot in my four years of college, and armed with an impressive resume I started "beating the pavement" just like the rest of my graduating class.

Eventually, I took my first salaried position with the LaGrange Area Department of Special Education, or LADSE. My supervisor there was a dynamic and professional woman by the name of Susan. Under her expert tutelage, I began the process of learning the ins and outs at LADSE.

Like every other company, corporation, or department, LADSE had its own way of doing things and I was eager to learn these "mysterious ways" as fast as I could. From clocking in to lunch breaks, from filing my W-2s to filling out forms for direct deposit, I soon learned that I had a *lot* to learn.

Professional work life was definitely *not* like college life. The hours were early and demanding, the pressure more real-life, and the coworkers and clients less forgiving. Like any recent college graduate, I felt inadequate and bothersome. And from the very beginning, I had to admit that things weren't as easy as I often made them seem to my friends and family, if only so they wouldn't worry about me.

From the start, I struggled with my appearance. I struggled with earning respect from my coworkers, peers, and especially my supervisors. I struggled with, well, everything!

I believe that my age had a lot to do with it. Despite my recent successes and the achievements I had managed despite my disability, I was still young. I had to learn to fit into a professional work environment, and I was slowly finding the challenge insurmountable.

But Sue mentored, tutored, and coached me as that all-important first professional year progressed. She helped me pick out clothes that were more professional looking, challenged me to have more empathy and understanding for my coworkers and peers, and helped me with various time-management issues.

Slowly, but surely, I made it through that first rigorous year of professional life. With Sue's help, I was able to look back on yet another accomplishment and be proud of myself and what I'd managed to do. But like so many of the other mentors in my life, I couldn't have done it without her . . .

THE LESSON

I learned many things that valuable first year in the professional workforce. I learned that there is a big difference between college and life. I learned that being cocky doesn't always work in your favor. I learned that I *don't* know it all. In fact, I learned that *nobody* does.

But more than anything, what Sue taught me was that, sure, your first year on the job is hard. Sure, you'll struggle with proper business attire. Sure, you'll struggle with fellow employees and earning respect. Sure, you're young and have a lot to learn. But don't blame it on your disability.

This was the most valuable thing I took away from the many invaluable lessons I learned that year, for it has truly stuck by me, even after all these years - and other jobs - later. Yes, I was disabled. Yes, I was having trouble on the job. But no, the one was not the cause of the other, and vice versa. In this case, 1 + 1 definitely did NOT equal 2.

Through her special way of tutoring and mentoring, Sue taught me that all recent college graduates go through a certain adjustment period. They're young, and they're cocky. They think they know it all, and they don't know the half of it. They're late, they're in a hurry, they're irresponsible, and they're inexperienced. Some of them have disabilities, some of them don't. It just comes with the territory.

Through her wisdom, she was able to at least give me some comfort throughout that torturous and trying year: The problems I was having were universal, they had nothing to do with my disability. While it didn't make the problems any easier to deal with at the time, it did give me hope for the future. After all, in time I would learn to dress better, be on time, be more polite, and learn the ropes.

If my disability wasn't affecting me then, it certainly wouldn't be affecting me later. And for that I was thankful. It gave me many things: Confidence. Relief. Perspective. But more than anything else, it gave me hope.

I wasn't alone in what I was going through. And neither are you . . .

JOURNAL ENTRY:

Has there ever been a time when you felt overwhelmed or unqualified? Describe this time in your life and how you finally coped with it successfully.

DON'T CONFUSE A CHANCE WITH A RISK

For someone who has been told what not to do all his life, hearing "don't" yet again was once too many. But when do you take a chance, and when do you take a risk?

It was a blustery Illinois night in the dead of winter and the weather report looked grim. But there I was, stuck at my college with a clear window of opportunity to drive home and sleep in my own bed, instead of in my cramped and stuffy dorm room.

I forget now what the reason for my being on campus that frigid winter night was. Either a meeting, or some preliminary registration duty I had to perform in anticipation of the coming semester. Either way, there was no urgency involved either way. Whether I stayed on campus overnight or returned home was of little significance.

Except to me, of course.

You see, my father called my dorm room just as I was preparing to leave for the 40-minute drive home.
"Rob," he warned. "The storm looks bad and it's only getting worse. Don't risk driving home tonight, stay in your dorm room. If things clear up, you can always drive home tomorrow. I'm warning you, stay there tonight and do not, I repeat, do NOT drive home tonight. We'll see you in the morning, son."

Well, that was enough for me. As someone who'd just heard "don't" one too many times in his life, I wasn't about to let a simple snowstorm bother me. I ignored my father's warning, nay, his demand, and walked right down to my car, got inside, and began driving home right away. I'd show him!

Instead, the snowstorm worsened. While I had heard various news reports (or were they just campus rumors?) that the storm was lightening up, it soon proved to be quite the opposite. My dad had been right, once again, and the snow came down in thickening drifts that soon made driving quite difficult, if not downright impossible.

Having just wrecked my own car a few days earlier, I tried to drive my mother's car even more carefully than usual. Still, the severe weather conditions soon proved too difficult and into a roadside ditch went my mother's car.

Not once, but twice. It even had to be towed out the second time!

By the time I finally got home that wild and windy night, my father was furious. Not because of the $600 repair bill I had just added to his already considerable burden, although that didn't exactly help matters much. Not because I'd disregarded his wishes, although that couldn't have helped things, either. But mainly because I'd confused taking a chance with taking a risk.

After all, what did I gain by coming home a night earlier? Not a thing. My safety was at issue, but instead of weighing the risks and getting all the information, I had simply driven home to prove a point. In short, I had taken an unnecessary risk.

There was no payoff. No great opportunity to overcome adversity. There was nothing essentially positive about the experience, save for the fact that I'd made it home alive. My father had warned me to stay overnight, based on information he had carefully recorded, knowing I was almost an hour away and wanting to give me the best information available.

Instead, I had ignored that advice and simply forged ahead, headstrong. I had confused taking a chance with taking a worthless risk. And I had lost.

THE LESSON

The difference between taking a chance and taking a risk is a very fine one. But I look at it this way: A chance offers more opportunity than failure, while a risk is just the opposite. The lesson to this story is this: Don't confuse a chance with a risk!

There was no reason for me to drive home that night. None at all. I was in no hurry. There was no dire need for my presence at home. No pressing deadline called, no great opportunity loomed. In fact, it probably would have been a lot easier to stay in my dorm room, snowstorm or no snowstorm.

The fact is, I was tired of people telling me what I could and, more often, could NOT do. "Don't" was the single word that stuck in my mind while I was driving home that night. As in the strict order my father had given me: "*Don't* drive home tonight."

There were several other words of his I should have listened to instead: Danger. Unsafe. Risk. But "don't" was the only one I heard. And that clouded my vision.

That, and the thick snow in my path. The thick snow my father had warned me about. But you don't need a snowstorm to tell the difference between taking a chance and taking a risk.

Surely there have been times in your life when an opportunity presented itself to you. A job. A class. An apartment. A friend. A spouse. Taking a chance at these opportunities is a worthwhile endeavor.

But what about the many risks one is faced with in their lives? Winning the lottery. Facing a dare. Beating the odds-or beating a dangerous snowstorm!

Time is too precious to waste on risking something out of spite, or anger, or stubbornness, or just plain folly. Chances must be taken in order to improve your life, succeed, or test your limits. But always, always weigh the options before pursuing a dream-or an opportunity.

It can make all the difference between taking a chance-and taking a risk!

JOURNAL ENTRY:

When was the last time you took a chance? How about a risk? Write about the differences between both, and describe a time when you confused the two.

GIVING TO RECEIVE

Learning how to give-to receive-is a valuable tool on your pathway to success. Want proof? Look no further than the book in your hands!

When I first began writing this book, I had high hopes and big dreams for its potential. After all, I've been wanting to write a book for years, decades almost. And here was my chance. Having a disability has not just made me "different," it has made me something else: special. Unique. One-of-a-kind. So I wanted to share what I've learned with others like me-in body, yes, but in mind and soul as well.

So even though some of the stories contained in this book were painful, and brought back ugly or hurtful memories, I wanted to get them down on paper anyway. It wasn't as easy as I thought, however.

Despite my advanced degree and personal, insider knowledge with every page you're reading, grammar and I have never exactly "gotten along." And combined with the usual typos and spelling errors of any rough draft, the first version of my manuscript contained the additional problems posed by my typing skills and the problems I faced because of my disability.

To get the book published, therefore, I knew I would need help. Professional help. Therefore, I began looking for a qualified editor to help me shape and mold my book into a polished project worthy of the nation's bookstore shelves. I began my search on the Internet, frequenting the many freelance writing and editing sites that flourish on the World Wide Web.

I eventually put an ad for the services I needed on several of these FREE sites, and in only a few short days got more responses than I could physically reply to! (I've since learned a new joke: "If you're lonely, just put an ad out for writers on the Internet!")

Narrowing the most qualified applicants down to a sort of "Top 10 List," I did some checking around on www.yahoo.com to research them all, finally narrowing this focused list even further: My Top 5. These people I Emailed back and forth, explaining my project, how many pages it had, the major problem, and asking how they could help. While all of these professionals were qualified, it soon became apparent that one, a former teacher and full-time editor, was the most qualified.

So, my "Top 5 List" was now down to one. But the biggest question remained: How much was this all going to cost me? Taking the time, energy, and creativity to write this book had already been a huge investment, not to mention printer, paper, and postage costs. Now I was going to have to pay someone to help me polish it off? I knew what I could afford, and couldn't squeeze much else out of my limited finances, so I knew it would be a struggle.

Not surprisingly, when my future editor sent me a sample contract, the price was way too high. Telling him so, this editor dropped the price considerably. Still too high, I told him so again. After much debate and friendly negotiation, we agreed upon a reasonable fee for my editing job. Yet I was hesitant to begin a professional relationship by "taking" so much. Instead, I wanted to give something back. And so, before he revised the contract one last time, I offered him, as a reward for slicing his prices not twice but three times, a small percentage of the profits should the book get published.

Surprised, the editor whipped up a new contract, royalty scale firmly in place, and emailed it to me overnight.

THE LESSON

While I don't recommend being a sucker, I do think it's important-even if it's not always good business-to be giving in your professional relationships. Not just because it's the right thing to do, but because it's also the right way to do business.

For instance, the editor I chose obviously wanted to work with me on this book. Not only was it personally touching to him as a former teacher to work with a "Special Ed success story," but he obviously wanted the job as well. And so, as a good businessman, he was willing to negotiate. Extremely willing to negotiate. And I could have simply taken his final offer and run with it.

But then I got to thinking: Is this the right way to start a long, prosperous, working relationship? After all, I want to write more books, and articles, and stories, for adults as well as kids. To find a reasonably priced, talented editor is not so easy these days, as I quickly learned. So why not stick with the right guy for the right price?

But how long would a talented editor want to stick around if all I did was take and take? And so I decided to give a little. And, since I couldn't afford to give any money in the present, I offered a percentage of what we might make in the future. This way, both of us stay motivated to make the best book possible, for as long as possible.

This way, we're in this thing together.
This way, we're not just strangers, we're partners.
This way, we have a common bond -a common goal - tying us together.
This way, we're in it for the long haul . . .

So the next time you find yourself dealing with someone,

either professionally or personally, take care to give a little now and then. It could just be the beginning of a long and glorious partnership . . .

JOURNAL ENTRY:

When was the last time you received something from giving?

PUTTING YOUR DISABILITY INTO PERSPECTIVE

Dealing with a disability is never easy. However, along life's pathways, we are often shown how good some of us really have it.

Growing up, I was always younger than the other kids in my Special Ed group on the campus of Illinois State University. To ease this minor setback, friendship was important. Luckily, I was presented with just such a gift in the form of Torrey.

My earliest memories of Torrey are of the two us hanging out together in the 3rd grade. So close were we, however, that our teachers encouraged us to branch out and meet new people. They soon got their wish. In the 6th grade, Torrey moved away to Montana and I was left to struggle alone without my best friend.

Fortunately, he returned just in time for our freshman year of high school! While we were never quite as close as those joined-at-the-hip years of good old elementary school, we were still blessed with a unique and inspiring friendship that has lasted to this day.

In fact, so close were we that when circumstances forced Torrey's family to move once again, Torrey actually asked my parents to let him move in with us so that he could finish high school with the rest of his graduating class. Unfortunately, my parents did not have the financial resources at the time to accommodate his wish, and Torrey did end up moving away after all.

To this day, my mother regrets this decision. For while I was able to graduate high school and move on to college, and eventually discover financial success, Torrey has just managed to "get by" with a series of minimum wage jobs.

Nonetheless, Torrey and I have kept in close contact over the years. This friendship never meant more to me than during 1997. This was one of the most difficult years of my life. I was having an increasingly difficult time at my job working for a well-known insurance company in their Aurora, Illinois service center. The pressure was intense and despite my best efforts on a daily basis, I was in very real danger of losing it. (Which I did in January 1998.) This would be a crushing blow to my financial independence, as well as my growing self-confidence.

In addition, I was extremely busy interviewing for other accounting jobs and attending a nightly study group for my all-important, upcoming CPA exam. Between the job pressures, financial worries, blistering pace, and lack of sleep, I honestly don't remember how I got through this time of my life at all.

Finally, after another long day at work, I went home to have a quick bite to eat and get changed for my CPA exam study group. Checking the phone messages, I heard a quick one from Torrey: "Hey, Rob. Can you call me? I need to talk."

Since it sounded like a normal message and I was already running late for my night class, I decided to ignore the message and go onto class. Later, during a much-needed study break, I called my Mom and asked if she had had a chance to speak to Torrey. In a strange voice, she replied that "yes, she had."

What I was to learn next was to change my life forever: Torrey had testicular cancer. My best friend was only twenty-five years old. And his cancer was so severe that within a week he was scheduled to go under the knife for an extremely risky procedure to remove the cancer and stop its progression into the lymph nodes-or anywhere else in his body, for that matter.

During that intervening weekend, however, I was able to shift my priorities and finally got to spend some quality time with my old best friend. During that weekend, the pressures of work and money- and even my own disability-took a backseat to the life-threatening nature of Torrey's condition.

Fortunately, after surgery and an intense regimen of chemotherapy treatments, the cancer was found to be completely removed and hadn't spread. Today, Torrey is back to leading a normal life and I am grateful for the good health of a man who is still my very best friend.

THE LESSON

What did that one glorious weekend spent with Torrey teach me? Lots of very different things, actually. It taught me to appreciate what I have. It taught me to slow down and smell the roses. It taught me not to underestimate the power of friendship. It taught me how to laugh again.

But more importantly, it taught me to put things into their proper perspective. So often in life we rush through our days, slurping down coffee in the morning, grabbing a quick bite to eat at lunch, and then stuffing our faces before collapsing into bed at night, exhausted. We can't believe it's already Monday morning again, but before we blink twice it's already Sunday night!

How many weeks do we spend like that? Rushing from Sunday to Monday only to start it all over again the very next week? How many months go by in that same manner? How many years? Spending that precious weekend with Torrey-a weekend that we both knew could have been his last-taught me to look around and see things as they really were. I eventually did lose the very job that was giving me such problems at the time, but having spent that time with Torrey made it all the more easy to cope with.

Everything was easier to cope with. My financial pressures hardly seemed significant in the face of Torrey's sickness, and neither did anything else for that matter. I was lucky to be alive-we both were-and complaining and griping about things we couldn't control wasn't doing either of us any good. It would have only wasted the precious few moments we thought we had left together.

Naturally, Torrey's recovery has only deepened our friendship and made me realize just how fickle life truly is. And as time has passed, I often find myself falling back into the same old "rush from Monday to Sunday" routine, complete with the same old job and financial pressures.

But they're not the same. Not really. Because that week with Torrey changed my life, and now I can finally look at things-in perspective!

JOURNAL ENTRY:

Ask yourself, "What if this were my last week on the planet?" Now, write about how you might view things differently if this statement were really true . . .

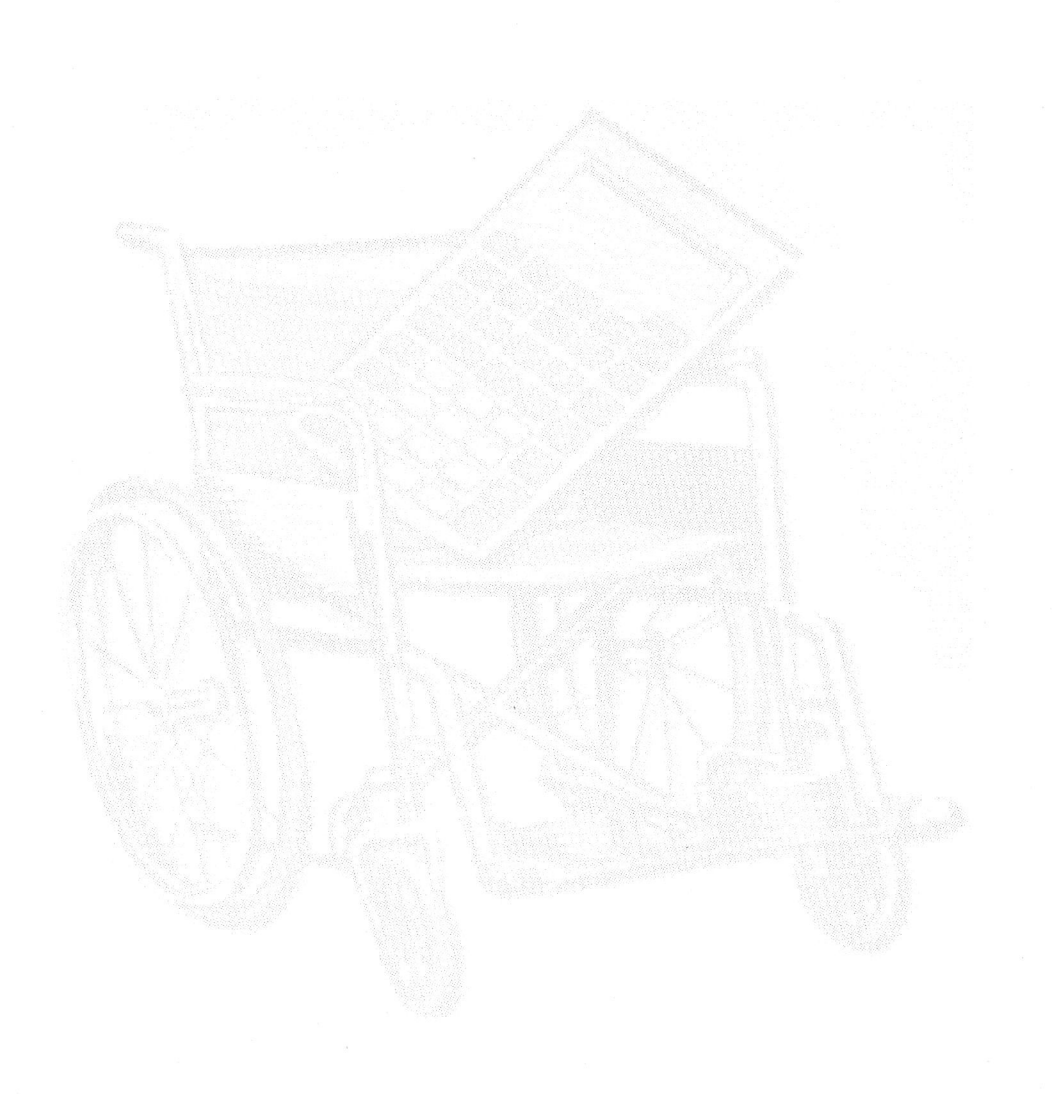

SECTION THREE:
QUAKE THE BARRIERS

QUAKE THE BARRIERS

If the barriers along life's pathways are what challenge us, delay us, discourage us, prevent us, and dismay us, then there's only one thing for us to do: Quake the barriers!

Quaking the barriers is different and unique for each of us. Some of us run and hide from the barriers that we daily face. For instance, if finances are an issue, we continue spending non-stop, ignoring those annoying calls from credit card companies and banks.

Some of us sneak around the various barriers in our pathways. Over the same issue of money problems, we may find ways to cut corners on the items we enjoy rather than giving them up altogether.

Others find ways to break down the barriers in our path, like so many bulls in a china shop. For example, in the same case of finances, some of us may simply take on an extra job to be able to afford all the wonderful things we want-and then some.
Still others find unique ways of beating their personal barriers. Instead of going without, spending less, or charging more, some of us may decide to take in a roommate, thus freeing our locked cash supply up for a little necessary spending.

Whatever your own personal style of "barrier quaking" may be, if it works for you, all the better. However, if you are having troubles knocking down, sneaking around, jumping over, or slipping under the many and various barriers along your personal pathway, enjoy the following stories, lessons, and journal prompts. They are all designed to help you quake those annoying barriers, either with the help of others, or all by yourself!

QUAKE THE BARRIERS...
WITH THE HELP OF OTHERS

SEEKING INSPIRATION FROM INSPIRING TEACHERS

I have had many teachers inspire me over the many years of my schooling, but few have touched me as much as Mrs. Quinn and Ms. Carver.

Teachers have a special place in the hearts of most people with disabilities. Since we are often relegated to self-contained classrooms, they are usually the one adult figure we spend most of our time with, often for over seven hours each and every day. Also, since several grade levels are occasionally placed in the same classroom, we regularly have the very same Special Education teacher for several years at a time, furthering our relationship all the more.

This can, of course, be a curse if you are stuck with a bad Special Ed teacher! (And I've had my share of those as well.) However, it can be a real blessing when you come across the likes of a very "special" Special Ed teacher like Mrs. Jill Quinn:

Jill, or "Mrs. Quinn," as I knew her back then, was my junior high school Special Education teacher. In a self-contained Special Ed classroom like the ones described above, I was with Mrs. Quinn for most of the day. It was a place for me to take tests and work on homework. And even though she went on maternity leave halfway through my 7th grade class, I know I'll never forget her for as long as I live.

On my I.E.P. for that year, or Individual Education Plan, which is required by Public Law 94-92 of the Individuals with Disabilities Education Act, or I.D.E.A., Mrs. Quinn stated that she wanted me to get at least a "B" in all of my classes.

I worked hard, but not hard enough in one class, where I learned I was earning a "D" and not a "B." Naturally, my parents were quite upset, not to mention Mrs. Quinn. As a result of what I had learned from my favorite teacher at the time, I quickly asked the teacher for any and all extra credit opportunities I could take advantage of. True to my IEP, I ended up getting a "B" in ALL of my classes that semester.

Thanks, Mrs. Quinn!

If Mrs. Quinn pushed me to achieve high standards, my last Special Education teacher, Ms. Carver, pushed me even more rigorously. Like Mrs. Quinn, my self-contained Special Ed teacher before her, Ms. Cheryl Carver was a truly great lady. In a word, she would not put up with any games!

If I thought Mrs. Quinn drove me hard in junior high, I still wasn't prepared for high school and the likes of Ms. Carver! However, her drive and determination soon wore off on me and I found myself reaching personal goals I had never even entertained before.

For one thing, Ms. Carver single-handedly helped me get better testing accommodations, study for, and take the ACT test, necessary for many college entrance boards. Not only that, but without her tireless effort and determination, I am quite sure that I would never have gotten into the University of Illinois.

But beyond the ACT and U of I, Ms. Carver pushed me personally as well. She helped me not just strive for personal and professional goals, but to form certain goals that I would have never even imagined for myself previously.

Without these two great teachers, not only would I not be where I am today, I wouldn't even be the person I am today . . .

THE LESSON

The many and numerous lessons both Mrs. Quinn and Ms. Carver taught me extended far beyond the reaches of their combined Special Ed classrooms. In fact, I have carried most of those very lessons with me throughout my entire life.

From Mrs. Quinn, I learned two things:

First, I learned not only to have respect for myself but to respect others as well. She taught me that disabilities were nothing to be ashamed of, but also that they were nothing to slow me down. Therefore, I could achieve anything anyone else could. That went a long way toward restoring my own self-respect.

It also helped me to see that there was no "us" and no "them," or people with or without disabilities. We are all the same, and we should all be able to get along-inside and out of the classroom.

Second, I learned to put forth the highest effort possible. Not just in the classroom, but outside of it as well. While her focus point for the year was to get a "B" in every subject, the lesson learned went way beyond good grades.

It taught me to strive for excellence in everything I did, all the time. Which is something all of us could use a little bit more of these days . . .

From Ms. Carver, I learned one very valuable lesson that has served me well throughout my life, and that was to not be content with where I was and to seek a higher level at all times. If I got here, that's fine, enjoy it, revel in it, be proud of it, but never, ever stop trying to go just a little bit farther and get there.

Then, when you're there, start the same process all over again . . .

JOURNAL ENTRY:

Who was your favorite teacher ever-and why?

VALUING FRIENDSHIP

Friendship is as hard to come by as acceptance, but occasionally you find both such prizes wrapped up in the very same package!

Who can say how a friendship really starts? One day you meet a delightful stranger, or perhaps even not so delightful. (After all, some of my best friends aren't all that easy to get along with! I bet this is true of some of yours as well.)

Somehow, somewhere, you end up having a pleasant conversation-or even a heated debate-over a quiet-or not-so-quiet-cup of coffee. Days pass, then weeks, then months, and before you know it, you have a friend.

Sometimes, you even come out on the receiving end with a "best" friend . . .

Such a delightful and happy "accident" happened to me when I was casually introduced to Khushnaaz.

I met Khushnaaz, or "Khush," as her friends call her, through one of those happenstance of people and places in all of our hectic lives. In college, I had a friend who was my RA, or Resident Assistant, in my dormitory, who had a friend who majored in Accounting and was roommates with my friend, Ruth. One day, by hook or by crook, Khush and I were finally introduced.

We've been friends ever since. Khush and her husband Zubin have an innate way of making you feel welcome, be it in their home or a crowded coffee shop or just passing on a busy street. They also have a way of making you feel important.

Through Khush I have learned the true meaning of friendship. As you have read in other stories, some of those I called my closest friends would go on to ignore me or, what's worse, betray me. Yet through thick and thin, Khush continues to inspire and comfort me through her undeniable and unconditional support.

Meeting, keeping, and holding onto friends isn't the easiest thing to do without a disability, but the challenges of keeping a friendship alive and thriving during the emotional and physical ups and downs of having a disability only serve to compound the every day problems.

Yet through it all, Khush has always treated me as her equal and I have never felt disabled in her presence. Her exuberance and positivity has further encouraged me to learn how to enjoy what I have in my life, in good times and in bad. Despite my loving family and numerous achievements, it always helps to have a friend in your corner, cheering you on and lifting you up when you feel down.

Khush is that friend.

Hopefully, Khush will always be that friend.

And knowing Khush, she always will be . . .

THE LESSON

Naturally, I have benefited from having a true friend like Khush. I encourage you to do the same. First off, however, it's always good to ask yourself a few questions:

Who are your acquaintances?
Who are your friends?
Who are your real friends?
Who are your best friends?

This isn't the kind of lesson that requires a pencil and a sheet of paper. You can usually tell instinctively who your real friends are, who are the hangers on, and who are mere acquaintances who wouldn't give you a dime to use the phone-let alone thirty-five cents! Seek out your best friends, and nurture that friendship as often as you can. Like a favorite plant, feed it with phone calls and surprise visits. Water it with pleasant surprises like thank you notes and unexpected gifts. Talk to it often, and weed out those unpleasant moments with frank discussions and, when necessary, heartfelt apologies.

Unlike your family, you actually get to choose your friends, so I encourage you to choose wisely. Your gut is often your best indicator when choosing a friend, as compared with your head or even occasionally your heart. For it's your gut instinct that allows you to trust someone completely, or turn away from them when those nagging concerns just won't go away.

Like finding a supportive group of professionals or a positive workplace, spending time with good friends, or even just one good friend, can be balm for your soul and a Band-Aid for your emotions. It is good to rely on yourself, but not all the time. And while a family member will often tell you something just because they think it's what you want to hear, it is often your best friend who will have the courage to play Devil's Advocate and tell you what they really think instead.

    This is invaluable as you amble down life's winding pathways. So as you do, make sure to take frequent pit stops to be with friends and fill up on their unending love and support.
You'll be glad you did!

JOURNAL ENTRY:

Write about one of your very best friends. What does this person's friendship mean to you? What does your friendship mean to him/her?

NEVER LOSE FAITH IN YOUR FELLOW MAN

For some, computers are a luxury. For others, they are a pathway to a modern technology that will knock down barriers at the speed of light. But only if you can afford one . . .

I realized early on that, no matter how hard I tried, my lack of handwriting would always be a barrier to my learning process. While my lively and creative brain could think up limitless imaginative stories, accurate answers, and potential solutions, my shaking hands had a bonafide problem with spelling them out on paper.

Despite my success as a mainstreamed student, the barriers thrown up by my lack of handwriting were threatening to send me straight back to the self-contained Special Education classes I was so intent upon avoiding.

As my frustration mounted and the school board plotted, however, a new invention was discovered that would soon change my life forever: The computer! Modern technology brought this gift to our school in 1984 and it was not long before my parents and I realized the impact this new technology would have upon my schoolwork.

With a computer keyboard, glowing monitor, and endlessly flowing printer, no longer would my shaking hands and completely illegible handwriting be an issue. With one wave of the magic wand known as "technology," a solution had appeared to one of my biggest barriers to a proper education.

Yet, as I've discovered on my own life's pathway, when one barrier falls, another one soon erects itself, often bigger and badder than the one it just shook down! In this case, the barrier to this new technology came in the form of money. As in, my family and I didn't have enough!

For months and months, as computer companies produced faster and smaller and, eventually, more affordable computers, they were still out of our reach. Working class people with strong hands and big hearts, my parents could still not afford a computer to solve my handwriting problem.

I took a typing class, paid for by my school, to prepare myself for the solution that I knew was just down my own personal pathway.

Eventually, over time, my parents were able to afford an almost prehistoric (by that day's standards) Apple II + computer, which included a monitor and keyboard. Finally, the faith I had had in my parents, and my future, had been rewarded.

Combined with my typing lessons I took in junior high, the computer, while big and bulky, old and slow, could nonetheless make my homework lessons a whole lot easier. Unfortunately, my parents were still not able to afford an all-important printer. Meaning that while my assignments may have been neatly typed, proofread, and resting inside my old Apple II + computer's hard-drive, I had no way of turning them in to my teachers!

Still, my faith remained strong. I had always triumphed over adversity before, both mental and physical, and I would again. As fate would have it, a local reporter decided to interview me about my determination to not only succeed, but excel, in the high school marching band, something unheard of in a person with CP. While it was an uneventful interview for the most part, toward the end my Mom happened to mention my need for a printer to go with my "new" computer.

Not one to whine or complain about my own personal problems, many of my closest friends and classmates did not know about my need for a computer printer. Certainly, my fellow members of the high school band had never heard me mention it.

But when they read about my printer plight in the local paper, they immediately sprang to action to help me in my time of trouble- without my knowledge, of course. Through personal donations and out of their very own pockets, my fellow band members managed to surprise me with a brand new printer in only a few short weeks!

And so, because of the faith I had in my fellow man, not to mention their good will and perseverance, I managed to solve the problem with my handwriting and now had the power to turn in legible assignments without the school board having to hire someone to do it for me!

THE LESSON

I learned a valuable lesson during the many bleak moments I had in my quest for a computer and printer to solve my handwriting barrier: Never lose faith in your fellow man.

Never underestimate the power of compassion. Don't let the bad news in the paper, the rude sales clerk, the bad waiter, the red tape, the corruption, and the apathy of many modern day citizens cloud the fact that somehow, somewhere, someone has the courage, the decency, and the heart to make your dreams come true.

Of the many barriers I've faced in my life, obtaining a working computer has been one of the biggest. From not having enough money for one to the one I finally got not being compatible with the rest of the computers at my school, my pathway to a solution to my handwriting problem was fraught with obstacles, some of them seemingly insurmountable.

Yet I always knew, deep in my heart-and also in the back of my head-that someone would help. Having a disability, especially one that is misunderstood by the majority of the people you come into contact with, often means relying upon other people for help.

This is something you must surrender to at times, but something you should never rely on totally. Having a disability is like walking a sometimes fine line between being dependent upon others, and being dependent upon yourself.

I wasn't asking for handouts, wasn't asking for charity. I didn't want anyone to do my homework for me, or for teachers to "cut me some slack" just because they couldn't read my handwriting. All I wanted for myself was an even playing field with the rest of my classmates and friends, and the new technology introduced by personal computers would provide me with that.

Because of fate, perhaps, and a few band members reading a timely interview in the local paper, I was finally afforded that golden opportunity. And I've never forgotten that. I've never forgotten the generosity, the privacy, the hard work, or the sincerity of my fellow band members.

But more than that, I've never forgotten the way they restored my faith in my fellow man during a time when it was being sorely tested. And that is what I'd like you to take away from this story.

People can be greedy, petty, mean, spiteful, jealous, hateful, cruel, and indifferent. They can be rude, little, evil, wicked, sinful, backstabbing, and conniving. This we know. This is not news. It happens in the business world, it happens in the church. It happens in colleges and high school and middle schools and elementary schools all over the world. It happens with strangers, it happens with friends, it sometimes even happens within your very own happy family.

But never, ever forget that people can also be kind, generous, heartwarming, touching, sincere, and helpful. They can surprise you.

They will surprise you . . . if given the chance.

All you have to do is let them . . .

JOURNAL ENTRY

Write about a time in your life when your faith in others was at its lowest ebb. Now write about a time when your faith in others was finally restored, and how that made you feel:

LEARN TO EXCEL WHERE YOU FEEL MOST COMFORTABLE

Finding someplace where you feel comfortable is a great discovery. But learning to excel there is a great lesson . . .

While I feel very proud to be an accountant, I must admit that in my chosen profession I face numerous roadblocks and barriers on a daily basis. From clients to coworkers, from technology to superiors, it is a constant struggle simply to perform my various job duties, let alone excel.

Not so in the National Speaker's Association of Illinois Chapter, or NSA of IL. This group has made me feel completely accepted and have been supportive of me beyond my wildest imagination. In doing so, they have taught me one of my most valuable lessons:

As a practicing public speaker honing my presentation skills for a career giving seminars, readings, and presentations, I joined the NSA of IL to increase my skills and associate with other professionals in this very challenging and unique field. On my very first meeting of the NSA of IL, a woman by the name of Barbara, approached me, introduced herself, and told me that she respected me for deciding to become a part of the Illinois Chapter.

Not only that, but she further offered to send me a videotape of a man named David Ring. David is another disabled speaker whose videotape helped me to gain confidence in, and acceptance of, my continuing role in the public speaking arena.

Not only was this videotape of David an inspiration, but Barbara herself is a very well-known speaker in the organization. To have her take the first step of introducing herself to me, at my very first chapter meeting nonetheless, truly made me feel welcome in this very challenging and unique place.

But Barbara was not alone. Taking her lead, other well-respected professionals in the organization also approached me and welcomed me to the NSA of IL. Yet these were not merely empty gestures. All of these influential and talented people simply wanted to let me know that I had made the right decision in my career path. It meant that they respected my talent, as well as my message. That has truly been an inspiration to me.

As I became a candidate of the NSA of IL and attended more and more meetings, the rest of the chapter has proved to be as professional, welcoming, and supportive as those members who had first approached me. As such, I felt more and more nurtured to branch out in my speaking career, take additional risks, and try new ways of speaking, rehearsing, or presenting.

The comfort zone provided by these warmhearted and professional people has truly given me a place to stretch out my wings and fly. In fact, a year after joining this influential chapter, I was approached by its former president and asked to sit on a prestigious committee for an entirely new program.

The name of the program was Fast Track and it was aimed at speakers who were just starting out. It was also designed to help us find at least 20 paid presentations, which would help us become a full member of NSA.

THE LESSON

This lesson is two-fold: First, learn to recognize where you feel the most comfortable. Is it with your friends? Is it at your school? Is it at work? Is it with your family? Second, learn to excel where you feel the most comfortable.

Whether it be your job performance, your academic achievements, or simply breaking new ground at home, don't let your disability hold you back from achieving certain goals or breaking down particular barriers, especially where you feel the most comfortable.

There is nothing wrong with branching out and trying new things. And, indeed, if there is a third part to this lesson, it is this: Learning to excel where you feel the most comfortable will eventually lead to you branching out and performing better where you don't feel as comfortable.

For instance, in the preceding story, I learned gradually to do more and more for myself, and the organization, as part of the National Speaker's Association of Illinois Chapter. I became more and more adept at what I was doing mainly because I was made to feel accepted, welcomed, and most of all, comfortable.

Finally, eight months after my very first meeting with the chapter, I was asked by the former president to sit on a committee for an entirely new program. In this instance, excelling where I felt the most comfortable led me to a position where I could try my hand at something new. In my opinion, the two went hand in hand and I certainly couldn't have done one without first doing the other.

In your life, too, learn to excel where you feel the most comfortable. Then learn from those experiences and build upon them to find the confidence, aptitude, or security to branch out and try new things where you don't feel comfortable.

In this way, your comfort level will increase ten-fold and you will eventually find more and more places where you do feel comfortable. Until, finally, you will become comfortable everywhere!

JOURNAL ENTRY:

Discuss a time, event, or place where you felt comfortable. How could you spend more time there? Why don't you?

QUAKE THE BARRIERS . . . BY YOURSELF

NEVER GIVE UP HOPE

Need a GREAT example of having faith and never giving up hope? Look no further than man's best friend . . .

One late Monday evening in September, no different from many other late Monday evenings I've spent in my life, I took my faithful dog Shelton out for a nice, long walk. Along the way, I thought I'd dump the weekend's accumulated trash in the nearby dumpster before letting Shelton frolic on his own.

After dumping my trash, I turned around just in time to narrowly avoid being run over by a pickup truck speeding through the condominium's parking lot! Unfortunately, Shelton was not so lucky-at the last minute I looked down to see his leash disappear under the truck's front tires!

Fortunately, the leash broke and a panicked Shelton ran off in a state of fear and shock. I had no idea how far his adrenaline-fueled legs would take him, but my guess was pretty far. Naturally, myself and a few of my close family and friends began frantically searching high and low for poor Shelton. But in the dark despair of a chilly September evening it was all I could do to see one foot from the next, and I was finally forced to give up and go home-without Shelton.

Over the next few days, I was lost without that dog. I suddenly realized how important "man's best friendship" was to me, and I resolved to do anything I could to find him. No matter what. My sister Janice even drove 150 miles to help me find Shelton! Unfortunately, all of our efforts were in vain. Day after day, out I went looking for poor Shelton. Night after night, back I came-alone. Somehow, I managed to make it through an entire week and was relieved when my parents finally came up for the weekend to visit me.

Their first priority-and mine-was to begin looking for Shelton anew. I had posted flyers with Shelton's picture, the date he was lost, and my phone number everywhere I could think of, yet even after a renewed search effort and several days with the flyers up, not a single person had called me concerning Shelton.

As the somber weekend drew to a close and my family prepared to leave, they did their best to prepare me for the inevitable: Shelton was lost and, after an entire week of no sightings, could quite possibly be gone forever. Though I, too, had conceded this fact in the back of my mind, I still held out hope that my best friend was safe and sound somewhere, missing me just as much as I was missing him.

To cheer me up and take my mind off of the unsuccessful hunt, my parents, my sister, and my future brother-in-law all took me out for dinner and were even planning on going to a movie afterward. Despite myself, I began to cheer up amid family and friends at the nice restaurant my parents took us to.

Still, something nagged at the back of my mind and, although I hadn't received a single message from my blizzard of flyers posted all around town, I called home after dinner-and before the movie-just on the off chance that someone had called me about poor old Shelton.

They had! The excited message said that a man had recently spotted a dog matching Shelton's description in the bushes not far from where the accident had occurred. The man felt that the dog would still be there-if we hurried. Alerting my family that we would be skipping the movie, we all raced to the location mentioned in the man's message and, like some frantic car chase scene out of a bad movie, screeched to a halt.

Before we were even able to retrieve our search supplies from my Dad's SUV, we heard Shelton's familiar whimpering from inside a thick wall of sheltering bushes. Believe it or not, there was Shelton, looking frisky and no worse for the wear.

In fact, he had managed to gain weight in the week we had been apart! How's that for a future contestant on the hit show, Survivor?

THE LESSON

What does this "feel good" story about a man and his rescued dog have to do with surviving disabilities with positivity? Well, a whole lot, if you actually stop to think about it.

Having Shelton around, I realized only after he was missing for a week, was an unusually comforting thing for me. I cherished his company more than I ever realized. I looked forward to his furry paws and good-natured barks each night when I returned home weary and battered from another long day at work.

Losing him, or even just the thought of losing him, even though it was for less than a week, was one of the darkest periods in my life. I had lost a true friend, whether he walked on two legs-or four. It didn't matter to me; a friend was a friend.

And during that whole, long week of tireless searching and daily disappointment, I never gave up hope. I never lost my faith that somehow, somewhere, Shelton was still alive and desperately waiting to be found by his Master.

Even when I knew the odds were more than against us. (What can I say, I am an accountant!) Even when I knew the numbers weren't stacked in our favor. Even when everyone around me, and even my own common sense, said that Shelton was gone forever, I couldn't give up hope.

And, finally, my faith was rewarded when Shelton was found, safe and sound, and even a few pounds heavier!

Isn't that a lot like living with a disability? Many days are dark and full of despair. Disappointment is our best friend, and follows us everywhere we go. But we can never give up hope, never lose our faith that somehow, some way, we will prevail. Despite the odds that always seem to be stacked up against us.

Fortunately, we have friends to help us along the way. Friends like Shelton, or even the human variety. Teachers to inspire us. Heroes to motivate us. We have dreams and goals and desires just like everyone else, and it's those same dreams and goals and desires that see us through the hard times, the tough times, the depressing times, the failures, and the disappointments.

Even on your darkest days, never give up hope. Never lose your faith. Because your own personal Shelton is just around the corner, whimpering in the bushes, and waiting for you to find him . . .

JOURNAL ENTRY:

Has there ever been a time when you lost all hope? Discuss that time, and what happened to turn you around . . .

BE A FRIEND TO YOURSELF FIRST

Friendship is important whether you have a disability or not. But learning to be a friend to yourself first was one of the greatest lessons I ever learned.

It was supposed to be a happy time for me: I was finally graduating from high school. All of the hard work I had put into achieving my goals and knocking down, leaping over, or moving around my particular barriers had paid off. Not only would I have an essay published in my class' graduation program, but I would be ending my high school career with a personal pride I had worked long and hard to achieve.

And so I was more than just a little excited as the week before graduation finally approached and my entire graduating class headed off for a relaxing day of class fellowship, good times, lifetime memories, and just plain fun. We were headed to a place known as Great America and Second City in Chicago, and as the bus headed toward our exciting destination I imagined the day ahead of me in my mind:

My closest friends and I would spend the entire day sharing experiences that would cap off a truly amazing year. The buddies I had enjoyed four long years with and I would walk everywhere together, eat together, experience everything there was to experience-together.

Arm in arm, we would laugh and tell jokes, lend each other money for stupid souvenirs we didn't need, and look back upon the last four years with fond memories and plenty of inside jokes to spare. And, when it was all said and done, our senior class trip would truly be a day to remember.

Yes, it would be a day to remember. But not in the way I first imagined:

Once the bus had arrived at its destination, I was surprised but not alarmed when my friends exited the bus rather quickly. More quickly than I. In their eagerness, I assumed that they had simply rushed to get off the bus without looking back. I was sure that they were simply waiting for me by the time I got off the bus. But when I emerged, my buddies, my padres, my companions, my "friends," were nowhere to be seen.

I had been ditched. On our senior class trip, no less. The day we had all been looking forward to for months, and that I had been planning so naively for weeks. I was left abandoned, disappointed, betrayed, and alone.

As I wandered around Great America alone, taking in the sights and occasionally running into a fellow classmate or two, I pondered the experience over and over again in my confused mind: How could my buddies do this to me? How could they ditch me like that? Were they even thinking of me as they wandered around, arm in arm, laughing and having fun? Had they ever cared about me at all? Had they ever truly been my friends in the first place?

What had started out as a day of fun and frivolity had turned into a depressing nightmare. I spent the day counting the hours and ignoring the sights, wallowing in my own despair and wondering how I could have ever been so stupid. When the day was finally over and we all returned to the bus, I found a seat far away from my "friends" and spent the ride home in silence.

"Happy Senior Class Trip" indeed . . .

THE LESSON

Being abandoned, misled, and betrayed by people you hold dear to you is a painful experience. Especially to a high school kid who was simply expecting a day of fun in the sun with his very best buddies. But it taught me one very important thing: If I was ever to be truly happy, I was going to have to rely on myself from now on.

In the end, it was one of the most valuable-and painful-lessons I have ever learned. After all, true friendship is born of more than mere convenience. The guys I had thought were my friends all along were merely acquaintances with something else on their minds. Who knew what their ulterior motives were?

All I knew was that, when the chips were down and I really needed someone to spend the day of the class trip with, they were nowhere to be found. Maybe they thought I would slow them down. Maybe they thought I would hamper their fun, or hold them back from going places they thought I couldn't go. Whatever the reason, they showed their true colors that day and I never forgave them.

I did, however, end up doing something better: I thanked them! After all, they had taught me to be a friend to myself first, and that was a lesson we all could stand to learn. Friends are nice to have, and the best of them are there for you when you really need them. I am not saying that friends aren't necessary. Not at all.

What I am saying is that you need to be your own best friend, first and foremost. Who knows you better than yourself? Who is with you, day and night, and never lets you down? Who has nothing to gain by being your friend, and everything to lose?

You do, that's who . . .

So, ask yourself: Are you your own best friend? Or do you

live to please others? Do you place value on your life according to what other people think of you? Do you wear what you wear because you like the clothes, or because you saw them on a friend? Do your friends color your value system, or what you feel about yourself?

We could all use a good friend or two, but more importantly, we could all stand to be a much better friend to ourselves-right now.

JOURNAL ENTRY:

Has someone you thought was a "friend" ever let you down? Write about the experience and how you learned to cope with it. Were you able to be a friend to yourself first?

PUT YOURSELF IN THE PATH OF LIFE'S LITTLE SURPRISES

It's always nice to get one of life's little surprises. But how are you ever going to be surprised if you don't put yourself in the path of one first?

It was my second year of being a part of the high school Speech team and my squad was finally competing in the last tournament of the season. Naturally, we had worked hard all year long to get to this point, and all of us on the team felt that we were ready.

We also felt that we'd never been so nervous! I was especially so, considering that at that point in my life simply qualifying for the High School Tournament of Champions would have been one of the pinnacles of my high school achievements, but first I had to win the Tournament in my event. Naturally, as we traveled by van to the nearby high school where the tournament was being held, there were more than a few butterflies riding along with us- inside our stomachs!

As the competition progressed, I was disappointed to learn that the individual speakers in my event, Extemporaneous Speaking, would speak on only one current event question, which was selected from three questions throughout the tournament. We usually prepared a different question each round from a choice of three. Although this option must have been quite simple and much more convenient for the judges, I felt that it did very little to enhance the competition of the actual speakers.

Still, as I have done so very often in my life, I played the hand I was dealt and simply tried harder than ever to make my speech as unique as it possibly could be. Everyone on our team who competed in my event eventually completed the exhausting rounds of public

speaking and, as we huddled nervously together in our seats awaiting news of the finalists, we were delighted to learn that all four of us in Extemporaneous Speaking were numbered among the total of six finalists! I was delighted to learn that I was one of them!
As we anxiously listened to the finalists' names being read after the final round, I mentally calculated the awards my teammates and I would bring home:

6th place was awarded to one of our teammates, Ruth. As the applause died down and the 5th place and then the 4th place winners were both announced, the fact that none of us were named made my team even more ecstatic. After all, that meant that the top 3 competitors were from our high school!

Nervously standing in front of the Awards assembly, I joined my teammates in listening as the top awards were announced. 3rd place went to Moria, while 2nd place was awarded to a dear friend of mine, Jennifer. I had never been so proud! As I congratulated her, I also realized that something contagious was happening throughout the crowd gathered around us.

As my teammates looked at me with pride shining through their eyes, I realized that the announcer was waiting for the applause to die down before announcing the last name. MY name! Yet, in anticipation of this event, the crowd could not contain their enthusiasm. Knowing the name that was soon to be called, they applauded more strongly than ever.

Friends and family certainly had reason to be filled with pride, as did I. But among the assembled crowd were strangers and audience members I had competed with all season. I was amazed when my name was finally called and the applause grew even stronger.

I had several reasons to be happy that day. Not only was the crowd's reaction to the judge's decision of my name for Tournament Champion reward enough in itself, but earlier I had been simply eager to qualify for the High School Tournament of Champions. But now I had actually won the tournament to qualify.

Talk about one of life's little surprises . . .

THE LESSON

Although becoming the Speech Tournament Champion was an especially pleasant surprise, I now realize that my actions put me directly in the path of that "surprise" in the first place.
After all, I had practiced hard, worked tirelessly in support of myself and my teammates, and done my best to be a winner in all areas of my life, not just as a productive member of the speech team.

I studied the other competitors closely, learned from my previous mistakes during earlier speech tournaments, never missed a speech practice, and always made sure to put my best foot forward every time I took to the stage. So perhaps becoming Tournament Champion shouldn't have been as surprising as it was.

This is a good time for you to examine the personal goals you have set for breaking down your own barriers along life's winding pathway. Are you putting yourself in the way of a few of life's pleasant little surprises?

Are you doing the work it takes to succeed? Are you acquiring the skills you will need to be successful? Are you taking time out to schedule, plan, and adapt to each and every hectic day? Are you letting your disability, whichever one it may be, get in the way of reaching your goals and living your dreams?

Surprises are something that happen to us because of direct actions we have taken, whether conscious or unconscious. In my case, I put myself in the path of my surprise by practicing hard, paying attention, doing my best, and believing in myself. Are you doing the same along your own pathway through life?

Why, even a really great surprise like winning a million-dollar lottery takes active participation on our part. After all, how are you ever going to win if you don't buy a ticket?

JOURNAL ENTRY:

Write about the last time you were pleasantly surprised by one of life's precious moments. Talk about how your actions helped to place you in the path of that special surprise.

MOST LIKELY TO SUCCEED

For two weeks every summer, at Easter Seals camp, I could go and lose my disability for a moment in time. But nothing lasts forever . . .

Like the rest of the kids in my neighborhood, I went to camp every year. For two weeks each summer, I attended Easter Seals camp. Here was a place where other kids like myself, and even disabled counselors, could gather and lose our disabilities for a moment in time.

When I was very young, and still learning to deal with my disability, Easter Seals camp became the one place I could disappear and not stand out. The one place where, among other special children, I could finally be "normal." I didn't have to feel out of place, didn't have to apologize for who I was, didn't have to make excuses or be embarrassed.

For two weeks a year, I was just like everybody else in the world. I could run and jump and play games and forget about the funny stares and awkward comments that filled my days back home. Camp was a haven, a safe place to be. But as I grew older, I knew that I couldn't just live for those two weeks every summer. I knew that I couldn't rely on egg races and specially trained counselors to make my life easier. As I grew as a person, however, camp began to hold me back.

I knew that, eventually, I would have to grow up in, and deal with, a modern world full of all kinds of people, and not just my family from camp and camp counselors. And so, gradually, over time, I began to view my time at camp just a little bit differently.

As I grew older, I wanted to take parts of camp home with me, to bite off and savor them for use throughout the year. I wanted to capture the feelings I had of being normal, and powerful, and most of all, happy. But how?

Before my very last visit to Easter Seals summer camp, I came up with a plan. I felt that I was not alone in my wishes to take camp home with me every summer and feel more capable and empowered throughout the year. I felt that something was needed to encourage my fellow campers to go beyond their disabilities, both at camp and after they returned home.
Beforehand, I got in touch with several counselors and the camp director and shared my plan. Having received permission to put it in order, I sent out a mailer to all the returning campers over thirteen, asking them what kinds of empowering activities they would like to participate in that summer. Gauging their responses, I had three plaques made.

These plaques represented awards. The first plaque was for the Volunteer Award. I felt that happiness was one thing, but helping to make others happy was even more important. And so I designed an award to present to the camper who participated in the most volunteerism at camp.

The second award was for Leadership. The criteria for this award was to encourage older campers to take charge and show some leadership among the other campers. I knew that the real world made success of its leaders, and that if campers could become leaders, why couldn't they do the same thing once they got home?

The third award was for Most Likely to Succeed. This award encompassed the many different areas needed to succeed, both in camp and the real world. Campers and staff were asked to vote on the one person whom they felt had all the qualities needed, not just to survive in the real world, but to SUCCEED.

The winner of the Most Likely to Succeed award that year was a young quadriplegic with cerebral palsy named David. Were his fellow campers correct in thinking David had all the tools necessary to succeed in the real world?

You be the judge: David recently passed the bar exam and is

now practicing law in Illinois.

THE LESSON

Success is measured by many things. You don't have to pass the bar exam and become a lawyer to be successful. You don't even have to go to college or finish high school. Many of today's most successful entrepreneurs never did either, yet their work has affected the way the rest of us live, work, and play.

Success is not measured by money or fame, houses or cars. Doctors and lawyers are successful people, but so are nurses and orderlies. So are the cleaning crew and trash detail. Success is an inner measure used by each of us in turn to decide what we'd like to achieve, and how far we can go to get there.

My own path to success is not finished. I have many more dreams and goals to obtain before crossing the finish line. This is likely to be the same for you. Whether your dreams are for financial success, starting a new business, or just getting a job and starting your own family, no one can determine whether you've won or lost in this magical game of life-except yourself.

Perhaps that is the lesson here. While only one person won the Most Likely to Succeed award my final year in camp, the idea was to inspire others to achieve more. I loved Easter Seals camp, but I didn't want it to end there. I wanted to remain positive and happy the rest of the year, and not just for two weeks. I felt that my fellow campers agreed with my philosophy and shared many of my own dreams and desires.

And so I thought of a way to cheer us all on, to make us think a little harder about our disabilities and go a little farther toward preventing them from stopping us from doing the things we wanted to do.

Things like volunteerism and leadership are qualities that

every person possesses, whether disabled or not. But sometimes we get so bogged down by life that we forget to lend others a helping hand, or raise a hand to be heard by others. My small awards ceremony and simple plaques were just one step toward making us go beyond our disabilities.

So what about you? Which award would you have won that year? Which award would you have liked to have won?

But more importantly, what could we all be doing now to win all three?

JOURNAL ENTRY:

Where is the place that you felt most special when growing up? Write about that place, and share why it holds a fond place in your heart. Have you found ways to push yourself and others to expect more from themselves?

ALWAYS WANT MORE

As you wind along the pathways of your life, continually stop and ask yourself, "Could I be doing more to make myself happy?"

Many people with disabilities reach a certain plateau and are satisfied with where they are. So satisfied, in fact, that they stop reaching for higher and higher levels of achievement. This is a story about how important it is that you always keep looking for that higher level, no matter what.

During my sophomore year in college, I was fortunate enough, or smart enough, to take a class in D-Base Computer Programming. While I found it both challenging and refreshing, many of my fellow students were severely taxed by the rigorous demands of this unique type of programming.

In fact, when it came time for a test, many of my fellow students studied 10-15 hours just to make a passing grade. Yet somehow I only needed to study for an hour or so for the same exam. (In the same vein, I somehow also managed to get an "A" on each of our tests.)

In fact, my class average was so high that by the time it was over, I was given the option of completing a special programming project in lieu of the regular final exam. A project I chose to do without hesitation, and one that would play a pivotal role in this story.

Around this same time, I got a part-time summer job at Burger King. The two worlds couldn't have been more different from each other. While I enjoyed my curriculum and naturally flourished at my programming class, I hated my fast-food job with a passion. The hours were long, the pay was low, and the menial labor did little to challenge or even stretch my vibrant imagination.

In fact, so loathsome was the fast food job that I sought other work, applying for an airport security position that would at least let me come home at night not smelling like a French fry doused in watery ketchup!

Unfortunately, the airport security job fell through at the very last minute and I was forced to labor away at Burger King until I finally looked around and thought, "I need something more." Instead of being down about the airport job falling through and toiling instead with the burgers and fries each night, I started looking at my options and wound up with a unique solution. Since I had excelled at the computer-programming class, and passed my final project with flying colors, I was able to find employment in that area. It was partly as a result of my frustration at Burger King, partly as a result of gaining so much confidence in my computer skills during the rewarding class time, but mostly because I never stopped asking myself, "Could I be doing more?" that I sought out, applied for, and finally got that programming job.

Not only did the new business opportunity pay a whole lot more than Burger King did, but much more importantly, it was a job that pushed me to constantly try harder, learn more, and excel.

THE LESSON

There's a famous line in the movie Wall Street where Michael Douglas's character is defending his hostile (takeover) actions to a large group of worried shareholders. The line? "Greed is good.". Only, that's not the "more" I'm talking about in this story's title.

The "more" in this case is different for every person, whether you're disabled or not. In my case, I wanted more personal and job satisfaction than just flipping burgers. However, for someone who's never had a part-time job or possibly any job at all, maybe their "more" would in fact be flipping burgers.

The fact is, we are all struggling just to move higher and higher up our own personal (fast) food chain. Whether or not we "make it" is irrelevant. The point is to always keep wanting more.

More for yourself.
More for your spirit.
More for your mind.
More for your soul . . .

Even if your dream job-your more-is in fact flipping burgers, don't be content with just flipping burgers. After all, once you've mastered the art of the greasy spatula, what's next? Assistant manager? There you go. Shoot for that. And then what? Manager of your own store? Regional manager of an entire district? Corporate manager in some big high-rise? Who's to say it will even stop there? Reach higher. Try harder. And don't be afraid to fail.

Always seek more out of your existence, be it flipping burgers, graduating from college, or just talking with your friends. Having a disability may prevent you from running a 4-minute mile or competing in the Olympics, but it should never dissuade or impede you from winning a gold in your own personal Olympics of life . . .

JOURNAL ENTRY:

Ask yourself, right now, "Could I be doing more?" And if so, what is the "more" you could be doing-and why?

PUTTING YOUR TRUST IN PROFESSIONALS

Having a disability means relying on lots of people-professional people. From doctors to lawyers, putting your trust in professionals isn't always an easy thing to do . . .

Like most of them, this book started out with a very different working title. You've heard me talk about barriers. You've heard me talk about pathways. You've heard me talk about "quaking" those barriers-knocking them down, going around them, or even over or under them.

So was it any surprise that the original, working title of this book was BARRIER QUAKE: "Shaking" Down the Barriers Along Life's Pathways? Not bad, huh? Having come up with it, and envisioned it, and pictured it, for several years before actually writing it, I was kind of partial to it myself.

And so how did it go from BARRIER QUAKE to FROM CP TO CPA? Well, it's an interesting story:

Having written a book, it was time to find an editor, a professional, someone to guide me through the ins and outs of the confusing-and highly competitive-world of modern publishing. Finding the right person was a real challenge, but I'm glad I did.

Not only were we able to fine-tune the manuscript itself, but I got some much-needed help in formatting the book to look better, chopping up the chapters into bite-size pieces, and using positive language as opposed to negative. I also got a concentrated list of publishers and agents to send the book to, which was almost as valuable as the editing itself.

I also got a first-class lesson in writing query letters and book proposals, two valuable tools necessary to help busy New York editors decipher which books to publish, and which to reject. Before my editor would help me send any out, however, he wanted to talk about the book's working title.

Since it was MY book, not to mention MY title, I listened with one ear open, the other definitely closed. Stubbornly, I knew what was best, and I had imagined this title for as long as I had imagined the book. But as I began listening, however, I heard some good points.

For starters, neither the words "barrier" or "quake" had anything to do with the subject matter of the book: Disabilities. In particular, cerebral palsy. My editor reminded me that there are only two or three opportunities for a bookstore shopper-and potential customer-to learn about your book in these busy days of scanning and browsing: The title, the subtitle, and the brief blurb on the back of the book.

The title, he said, was the key. The subtitle could help, but the title had to be a clincher. Not only for potential customers, but for potentials agents and publishers as well. And so, after much listing and going back and forth, we came up with the title you have in your hand: FROM CP TO CPA.

I like it. What about you?

THE LESSON

While I have been called many things, "stubborn" is not one of them. However, this book was a very personal project for me. The result of an almost thirty-year odyssey that has taken me from infancy through Special Ed classrooms, from self-contained to mainstream, from high school to college, from Driver's Ed to the open road, from not being able to write to learning how to type, and over and above any of my own personal expectations.

So messing with the title of my book was a big "no-no" to me. However, in between the heated discussion I was having with my editor, and several trustworthy family and friends and mentors and other professionals, I realized that I was paying this professional to do a job for me. If he had been paying me for my accounting services, I would expect him to listen to me. So why wasn't I showing him the same courtesy?

A professional, I was paying him not only for his services, but for his advice, his experience, his expertise, as well. And so I gave over and listened to him, point by point, blow by blow. And, once my defenses were down and I could see things objectively, I realized that by using the FROM CP TO CPA title, we could serve two purposes. Not only would I draw curious bookstore browsers in with a catchy title, but I could help educate the public by using the words "cerebral palsy" in the book's subtitle, thus schooling them in the fact that CP does stand for cerebral palsy, something many people in the "normal" world don't know.

There were other benefits as well, and I'm glad you bought the book. Now you can discover them for yourselves . . .

The point is, however, that when people with-and without-disabilities pay a professional for his or her services, they should listen. Pay attention. Examine thoroughly the pros and cons. Most importantly, be trusting. Trust a professional's judgment-not blindly- but instinctively. If it makes sense to you, don't second, third, or fourth guess it.

Go for it. I did!

JOURNAL ENTRY:

Discuss a time when you had to place trust in a professional- despite your better instinct. How did it turn out? How could it have turned out differently?

CONCLUSION:
HONING YOUR SKILLS-FOR LIFE!

In Professional Speech, just like in life, you need finely honed skills to succeed . . .

In March of 1998, I walked unannounced into the bustling Speech office at the College of Dupage and told the Director of Forensics, Steve Schroeder, that I would like to coach. Unfortunately, as spring was currently winding down on the wall calendar as well as the collegiate one, so was the competitive speech season.

"I'm sorry," said Steve. "We don't need anyone right now. Why don't you try back in the fall?"

Several long months later, when fall was finally in the air and I figured enough time had gone by, I got back in touch with Steve and reminded him of our conversation.

Remembering me from my own Speech days, when Steve had himself judged me, this time he said, "Yes."

For my first assignment, I was given the task of coaching Matt, a young sophomore. I worked with Matt briefly, due to the time constraints of the fast-paced Forensics season. In that time, I did my best to instill in Matt the basic skills and concepts of public speaking, as well as a few insider tricks I'd learned during my own duration on a college Speech Team. Together, we practiced religiously for an entire week. Despite the short time frame, I believed I did a thorough and inspiring job of coaching Matt. He did, too.

Apparently, we weren't alone in this belief. At the following week's Speech Tournament, Matt actually won the event I had coached him in, Impromptu Speaking, which just happens to be one of the most difficult and challenging competitions in the entire Tournament!

I was impressed, Matt was impressed, but most of all, Steve Schroeder was impressed. The very next week, he gave me a new student to coach, another young sophomore by the name of Jake. Apparently on a hot streak, the same experience I had with Matt repeated itself with Jake. After only a week's worth of rigorous coaching, Jake went on to win his chosen competition in his very first college-level Speech tournament.

I later learned that Steve had told both boys that he had found a phenomenal new coach to work with them. Excited, both boys were still somewhat skeptical upon first meeting me. They didn't know whether to think Steve was just being nice to a man with a disability, or whether I truly had the goods to deliver upon my fabulous introduction! After their impressive performance at both speech tournaments, the boys were no longer surprised.

Still, Jake was just a little more than hesitant as our first week together progressed. However, I was able to win him over by accepting a challenge to give an impromptu speech presentation myself! After witnessing my speech, utilizing the same precepts I was currently teaching Jake, he had no further questions about my ability - to coach or to speak!

As the season progressed, both Jake and I recognized his flair for Impromptu speaking, which involves little planning and lots of thinking on your feet! Not everyone has a knack for this challenging type of Forensics, but I sensed in Jake that he did, and his win in his first big tournament clinched that fact-for both of us.

Adding to his natural talent, Jake made it a practice to study quotations and practice sample Impromptu speeches based on those quotations from far and wide to increase his repertoire. This helped him immensely because the typical Impromptu speech consists of a mystery quote received by the speaker, only minutes before his speech, which he must translate into a six minute performance.

Along with practicing with these quotes, Jake began soaking up the skills, ideas, and concepts I taught him and began to hone them and develop them more and more-on his own. I could see it in his weekly performance, improving almost by the day. More and more, I saw those same skills, ideas, and concepts creep into Jake's speeches. I must admit, it filled me with pride.

As March wore on, Steve Schroeder and I decided to put Jake in the State Impromptu Competition. While Steve and I had high hopes for Jake, and indeed, Jake had almost as much confidence in his newly-acquired skills, we were all surprised when Jake took straight wins in each and every one of the Impromptu Rounds at the State Competition.

This was amazing on so many levels, both personal and professional, but primarily for two specific reasons. First, Jake was coming from a community college and it was literally unheard of for a community college student to make it all the way to the State Tournament Four Year Final Round, let alone win it! Second, Illinois is one of the toughest states to compete in for Speech, with all of its powerhouses in the highly competitive field of Forensics. Jake had truly gone up against some of the toughest competition in the country and not just held his own-but won!

Needless to say, his coach was very, very proud!
And, of course, I would love to take all the credit for his stellar performance. I would love to say that it was my influence that helped Jake win the tournament. I would love to say it was my tutelage that brought him this far. I would love to say that it was those skills, ideas, and concepts I had taught him that had made all the difference in the world!

I would love to say all those things, but I can't . . .

Oh, I know for a fact that I helped. I know I contributed. I know that, in many ways, Jake might not have been able to come so far so fast without me. But it was Jake who won the tournament. It was Jake who took home all those medals. And it was Jake who deserved them. Each and every one . . .

And here's why:

Sure, I may have taught Jake the skills, ideas, and concepts he needed to succeed, but Jake was the one who listened. Jake was the one who paid attention. Jake was the one who took notes, studied hard, showed up for practice, gave his all and, as a result, took home the prize.

Jake didn't just listen to those skills, ideas, and concepts I taught him, he took them and made them his own. He personalized them. He owned them. But more than that, he honed them. Developed them. Tailored them for his own personal use in his own personal situation to attain his own personal goals, hopes, and dreams.

Alone, I could have never instilled that personal desire in Jake. Alone, I could never have drilled in the drive and dedication and practice it took to achieve his personal dreams. Only Jake could possess that inner drive, and only Jake could go for it. And go for it he did.

And that is why I chose to use Jake's inspirational story to end this book. The message here is clear: I am only an author. I am only a speaker. In a way, I am only a coach. You can choose to do one of two things with my message:

1.) You can take my ideas, apply and develop them in your own life, and benefit from them.

2.) Or, you can forget about them and keep doing things the way you always have. In other words, "If it ain't broke, don't fix it!"

But whether you use the skills you learned in this book or those that you heard from a speaker or learned from a class, the end result is the same: The only way you can really improve your life is by finding specific skills and developing them to your own personal hopes, dreams, and desires, just like Jake did.

In other words, I can only "coach" you so far. I can only provide the skills, ideas, and concepts you need to succeed. The rest is up to you . . .

AFTERWORD:
What's Next?

Rob Pritts is not through achieving his life's goals and ambitions. In fact, FROM CP TO CPA is just the beginning. In spreading its message across the country, Rob is quickly gaining notoriety as a thrilling and popular motivational speaker. Corporate and non-profit groups alike are eager to hear his inspiring message, and practice the growth exercises introduced in the book.

As for future books, Rob plans numerous sequels to FROM CP TO CPA, this time containing YOUR stories. Rob knows that he is not alone in dealing with a disability, and that others are eager to share their stories as well. Future volumes in the CP TO CPA series will include personal and inspiring tales of people with disabilities from all over the country. To contribute YOUR story today, go to Rob's Website at http://www.cptocpa.com.

Finally, Rob's personal plans include spending more time with his friends and eventually getting married. Those who know him best are confident that Rob will accomplish all of his goals, and many, many more . . .

To order additional copies of CP to CPA!

Online Orders:
Please visit: www.mypublishinghouse.com

Postal Orders:
Weyant Press, Inc.
27765 McKee Road
Toney, AL 35773 USA

Please send me:

____ copies: **From CP to CPA: One Man's Triumph over the Disability of Cerebral Palsy** By Robin Pritts ($11.99 each + $3.95 S/H)

Ship To:

Name:_____

Address: _____

City: _____ State/Province:_____

Zip/Postal Code: _____ Country: _____

Telephone: (____)_____ Email: _____

Please add 8% sales tax to books shipped to Alabama addresses.

Payment:

___ Check Enclosed   ___ Money Order Enclosed
For credit card orders, please use our secure online processing agent at www.mypublishinghouse.com

Printed in the United States
825600001B